T0073624

WE THE SCIENTISTS

WE THE SCIENTISTS

*How a Daring Team of
Parents and Doctors Forged
a New Path for Medicine*

AMY DOCKSER MARCUS

RIVERHEAD BOOKS
NEW YORK
2023

RIVERHEAD BOOKS
An imprint of Penguin Random House LLC
penguinrandomhouse.com

Library of Congress Cataloging-in-Publication Data

Names: Marcus, Amy Dockser, author.
Title: We the scientists : how a daring team of parents and doctors
forged a new path for medicine / Amy Dockser Marcus.
Description: First edition. | New York : Riverhead Books, 2023. |
Includes bibliographical references and index.
Identifiers: LCCN 2022023324 (print) | LCCN 2022023325 (ebook) |
ISBN 9780399576133 (hardcover) | ISBN 9780399576157 (ebook)
Subjects: LCSH: Niemann-Pick diseases—Treatment. | Rare
diseases—Patients. | Genetic disorders in children—Patients—Family
relationships. | Parents of children with disabilities.
Classification: LCC RJ399.L95 M37 2023 (print) | LCC RJ399.L95 (ebook) |
DDC 618.92/0042—dc23/eng/20220802
LC record available at https://lccn.loc.gov/2022023324
LC ebook record available at https://lccn.loc.gov/2022023325

Printed in the United States of America
1st Printing

BOOK DESIGN BY MEIGHAN CAVANAUGH

In memory of my mother, who led the way

For my father, who kept us going

And for Ronen, who pushed me up the hill

All crises begin with the blurring of a paradigm and the consequent loosening of the rules for normal research . . . And all crises close in one of three ways. Sometimes normal science ultimately proves able to handle the crisis-provoking problem despite the despair of those who have seen it as the end of an existing paradigm. On other occasions the problem resists even apparently radical new approaches . . . Or, finally, the case that will most concern us here, a crisis may end with the emergence of a new candidate for paradigm and with the ensuing battle over its acceptance.

—Thomas S. Kuhn
The Structure of Scientific Revolutions

CONTENTS

INTRODUCTION:
WE THE SCIENTISTS

The early 2000s marked a hopeful time for many cancer patients. Decades of basic research, growing understanding of the biology of cancer, and billions of dollars of government investment had finally yielded breakthroughs in treatments. Targeted therapies homed in on specific proteins in tumors, stopping them from growing and spreading without many of the debilitating side effects associated with traditional chemotherapy regimens. New drugs continued to come on the market. Growing numbers of people started wrestling with what it meant to live with cancer as a chronic health condition rather than as a death sentence. As a reporter on the health beat, I spent a year working on a series of articles for *The Wall Street Journal* chronicling the transformation in cancer patients' lives. I came away from my reporting hopeful about what the new therapies could do.

Then, after finishing that series of articles in 2004, I got a very personal reminder of just how far we still had to go in finding effective treatments for cancer. In December of that year, my mother was rushed to the emergency room, doubled over in excruciating pain. Doctors diagnosed metastatic gallbladder cancer, a rare disease that, along with cancer of the nearby bile ducts, affects about 12,000 Americans each year. In comparison, more than 290,000 Americans are diagnosed with breast cancer every year.

I soon learned what that disparity meant. Those promising targeted therapies I had been writing about weren't available for people like my mother. That's because the pharmaceutical companies that run most of the clinical trials for new drugs weren't working on developing new treatments for gallbladder cancer; the market was simply too small to justify the resources and investment required to identify, test, and get novel drugs approved. Even if they had been willing to try, studies indicated that the time from a promising idea in a lab to market approval was closing in on seventeen years—far too long to ever help my mother, since people with metastatic gallbladder cancer rarely live more than two years. The only available options were drugs that over the decades had exhibited only limited success; the odds of them helping now weren't good.

At major cancer centers like the one where my mother underwent chemotherapy, there wasn't a lot of data available on how previous patients fared or if one drug seemed better than another. The number of patients with gallbladder cancer at individual institutions was in the single digits, too small to be statistically meaningful, and the researchers didn't pool data with all the other centers that also saw gallbladder cancer patients. Researchers who generated a hypothesis struggled to get funding from either the government or large private foundations to test their theories; as a result, promising ideas languished. Scientists interested in finding drugs for rare diseases often have to go it alone, with predictable consequences for patients like my mother. Each round of chemotherapy failed to stop or slow down the insidious progress of the disease. My mother died in May 2007, a few weeks after her sixty-fifth birthday.

After her death, a feeling of helplessness profoundly shook me. I had been reporting on promising new options for cancer treatments, but in my mother's case, we had none. Why? My mother's oncologist was thoughtful and compassionate but lacked any data upon which to base trying a different approach than one that had been failing for decades. A scientist I interviewed who was interested in pursuing novel research had collected gallbladder tumor samples, but they remained locked in a freezer because he couldn't get the time or funding to move the project forward. I felt I shared a portion of the blame too: Could I have done something different or something more to save my mother's life?

I started reading histories about successful patient advocacy movements started by patients with HIV and breast cancer who founded new organizations and confronted the medical establishment. I was struck by how many of the participants framed their efforts to accelerate drug development as part of a broader social movement fighting for social and political equality. In addition to helping drive the development of drugs in their own diseases, they tried to influence national health policy. HIV activists pushed the U.S. Food and Drug Administration (FDA) to think differently about the way it went about assessing if a drug was working. They wanted the agency, when weighing clinical trial results, to formally authorize the use of surrogate markers, data points that indicate patients are benefiting but don't definitively show they are living longer. The agency agreed and initiated the Accelerated Approval Program that over the years has allowed for faster approval of drugs for HIV and other life-threatening conditions. Breast cancer, disability and mental health activists, and other patient-driven groups also insisted that they should have the right to help shape policies surrounding clinical trials, including determining how much risk they were willing to take when trying experimental drugs. As a result of their activism, hospitals and academic centers routinely include community participants as members on institutional review boards that ensure the protection of the rights of people participating in research. Patients serve on various government advisory committees, offering their views on proposed projects or weighing in on some funding decisions.

But despite these important gains, my family's journey revealed to me that something larger wasn't working. Patients on government advisory committees are usually outnumbered by scientists and researchers; their presence can often seem more like tokenism than something transformative. One study I read discussed how even in partnerships explicitly set up to encourage collaboration, doctors, not patients, dominated the discussions and set the priorities. The concerns of patients too often remain on the edges of the scientific enterprise, rather than at its very center. While individual patients or groups successfully mobilized and achieved some victories at the edges, the heart of the system remained largely unchanged.

Science involves designing experiments, gathering data, and interpreting results. But none of these things take place in a vacuum; every step is shaped by value judgments made along the way. The questions investigators ask, the diseases they study, the trial design they choose, and the funding they receive encompass and reflect scientific reasoning but must also go beyond it. Scientists bring to all these things their personal backgrounds and experiences, aspirations and emotions, along with pragmatic assessments about what's already known about a disease and philosophical approaches about what's best for the common good. When only one group is given the power to gather, analyze, and interpret the data, it can skew the interpretation. Science is inherently a social enterprise, yet too often scientists operate behind closed doors, removed from the very people they intend to help.

In the months after my mother died, I began traveling around the country, supported by a health policy research grant from the Robert Wood Johnson Foundation. I wanted to meet people who were trying to change the current system. A few months into the project, a policymaker who had given me helpful advice about researching my mother's condition reached out. He told me about a fatal genetic condition known as Niemann-Pick disease type C (NPC) that mainly, but not exclusively, strikes children. The disease, which causes cholesterol to accumulate in tissues in the brain and other organs, was very rare, I soon discovered—only about two hundred cases were known in the US at the time, with an estimated five hundred around the world. Children typically appeared normal at birth, but then progressively, and inexorably, lost the ability to walk, talk, and eat. Most people diagnosed with NPC in early childhood were dead by the age of nineteen. There was no cure—but that wasn't the end of the story. Frustrated by the same feeling of helplessness that gripped my family after my mother's diagnosis, a group of parents whose children all had NPC had decided to take matters into their own hands.

Intrigued, I started talking to the parents, and I soon realized that they had embarked on a remarkable social experiment, one that had the potential to transform how we pursue cures for rare diseases and contribute to the creation of what one of the scientists who later joined the effort described as "the new paradigm," where patients and scientists are equal partners.

Ordinary people with no scientific background were not willing to leave science to the scientists. A movement was growing, empowering patients to gather and analyze their own medical data. These people called themselves "citizen scientists," and they used the internet to find one another. Some sought genetic information and test results—information they received from new direct-to-consumer genomics companies such as 23andMe and then shared with other like-minded patients in chat groups or organized communities springing up on Facebook. Others devised experiments, asking the kinds of questions that often didn't get attention from professional scientists because they were on topics or issues unlikely to lead to published papers in scientific journals, the process of which was an essential part of advancing scientific careers. In some instances, wealthy individuals or patients directed money to scientists but with one big condition: investigators could no longer hoard data. Researchers who might have once preferred to wait until a paper was published now met frequently to share and discuss their findings with one another and their benefactors. Science, and the notion of who was a scientist, was starting to change.

The parents I got introduced to that year knew their children didn't have a lot of time. As each month and year went by, their children lost more neurons and their cognitive abilities and motor skills declined. The urgency of their search for a cure was greater than that of the scientists who were also working on the disease, because they were racing to save people they loved. Although they weren't trained scientists, these parents wanted to produce scientific knowledge. From the outset, they had shared their children's medical records, read and discussed scientific papers, and held weekly conference calls in which they listed and prioritized promising treatment leads. They knew what they were doing was valuable; they studied *people*, whereas the scientists studied cats and mice. They also recognized there would never be a treatment in time to save their children if things stayed the same. And so, remarkably, they had convinced a few scientists working on the disease to forge an unusual collaboration with them in search of a cure.

. . .

UNTIL THE LATE NINETEENTH CENTURY, there were no professional scientists. Science was pursued by anyone with curiosity, intense passion, or personal interest in a topic. People built telescopes to identify planets or set out on perilous voyages of discovery around the world to gather and study interesting biological specimens. Such efforts were almost always funded by a personal fortune or the fortunes of others who shared common interests and goals. In the twentieth century, however, the notion that anyone could be a scientist gave way to the establishment of a profession. Science became a guild. To get in, you needed years of study, the acquisition of expertise, specialized training under the tutelage of seasoned veterans, and a university degree.

Over time, scientific projects got more complicated, and more expensive, to run. Governments stepped in, providing grants to fund research. As stewards of public monies, they required that recipients demonstrate some sort of sanctioned expertise. Professionals directed the studies, evaluated the utility of the projects, gathered the data, and analyzed and published the results.

Scientists still needed help from wider society. For one thing, they wanted patients and families to lobby Congress for more government funding to support basic science and advocate for bigger budgets for agencies that gave research grants, such as the National Institutes of Health. They needed patients to enroll in the clinical trials they organized, and to donate blood, tissue, and other samples to help advance their research, which revolved around questions they found the most interesting.

In a few cases, members of the public still played an important role in the scientific enterprise. In 1899, Frank Chapman, an ornithologist, organized the famous Christmas bird census, a one-day event in which amateur birdwatchers make observations and pool them for science—an event that still happens today, sponsored by the Audubon Society, and involves more than sixty thousand people. But that effort, along with similar ones that relied on citizens to report water levels in backyard streams or identify stars in the sky, were still largely directed and managed by professionals, who considered the data theirs and might keep it to themselves until they decided to publish. Scientists and amateurs were not equal partners in these enterprises. The scientists called the shots.

There were efforts from the very beginning to bridge the growing gap and retain public support. Annie Alexander, an amateur naturalist and heir to a shipping and sugar fortune, founded the Museum of Vertebrate Zoology in 1908. The Berkeley, California, museum, located far away from the center of professional activity in the field on the East Coast, depended on ordinary people to share their fossils in order to build its own collection. Annie hired a scientist, Joseph Grinnell, to run the museum in a way that engaged the public while still ensuring the credibility of the burgeoning collection among the established professional biology community.

Joseph took a hybrid approach. He knew there was a core set of information sought by professionals to enable their detailed analyses. So he developed a standardized, accessible method for labeling and collecting specimens that didn't require a degree in zoology to follow. Joseph understood that all the different individuals involved in supplying the specimens—amateurs and professionals alike—didn't have to agree on how to interpret the information. The data could still "have different meanings in different social worlds," wrote the scholars Susan Leigh Star and James R. Griesemer in a paper about the museum. But the standardization of the collection methods, the authors wrote, "provided a useful 'lingua franca' between amateurs and professionals" and opened up a way for them to identify common areas of interest, such as land conservation in California.

"The creation of new scientific knowledge depends on communication as well as on creating new findings," the authors pointed out. Amateurs and professionals do not have to reach consensus on every aspect of an endeavor in order to productively collaborate, the authors concluded, a lesson that is as relevant today as it was back then.

. . .

WHEN I FIRST BEGAN REPORTING on the NPC project, I could see the parents and scientists were trying to construct a fundamentally new kind of collaboration. They were good people who all wanted to save the children's lives. But despite their common goal, it quickly became apparent that they had different attitudes and approaches toward the production of science. For over half a century, the focus in medical research had been on discovery launched by an individual investigator and experiments inside a lab. The parents tried to force the lab doors open. They didn't intend to follow the usual rules.

The parents and the scientists I met had a list of leads to test. Some involved compounds that the parents could buy on their own and try on the children, without the scientists' approval. From the beginning, this created tensions. Was it truly a partnership if the parents used the scientists' data without permission to choose drugs to test on their children? Who exactly should decide how soon experimental drugs that were promising in animals but whose toxic effects were not yet fully understood should be tried in humans—particularly children who were unable to make their own decisions? How was it possible to accommodate the understandable desire of parents to save the lives of their own children without addressing the possibility that something could go wrong, which could in turn derail the prospects of future access to promising, potentially life-saving treatments for everyone else? The parents wanted to prioritize what they saw as in the best interest of their own children, without harming others in the group. The scientists, for their part, felt a moral obligation to the broader community, especially to patients who hadn't even been born. The parents and scientists were working together, but they also had fundamentally different interests. So when moral conflicts arose in their collaboration, I wondered, what ethical framework could be used to assess and resolve them?

These were new and difficult questions. It wasn't only the science that was inadequate in this situation, I realized. The system of research ethics that had evolved over decades to protect human subjects didn't seem to apply.

Existing rules, frameworks, and guidelines were not relevant to the new kind of relationship the parents and scientists were pursuing. The people who wrote the guidelines never expected parents to drive research, organize their own experiments, or work as partners with scientists. Many questions were unanswered because they had never been considered.

The rules were set up to protect vulnerable people from the scientists, doctors, and investigators, groups that had more power and more information than patients or families.

But when the parents themselves helped design and run the experiments, were they vulnerable? When the scientists insisted that the only valid and ethical form of scientific research was the gathering of data to benefit future, not current, patients, did this truly live up to the ethical ideal of justice? Both sides in the collaboration raised hard questions. But current ethical standards didn't recognize those questions, let alone try to solve them. Often, the disagreements over science seemed to me to primarily be disputes about values. This was fraught but absolutely fascinating territory.

WHEN I BEGAN THIS PROJECT, more than a decade ago, I could not be certain it would become a book. For years, I pursued it on the side, on weekends and in between my other reporting assignments, compelled to learn more. But the more I immersed myself in the subject, and the better I got to know the people and issues involved, the more I grew convinced that I was witnessing something potentially transformative. In 2012, I told my editors about the research I had been doing, and they encouraged me to write about it at length.

So began what would become, in 2013, a series of ten articles published in *The Wall Street Journal* about the parents and scientists whose efforts to work together and co-create scientific knowledge I had been following. I wanted to tell the story of the collaboration from both sides, and to start examining the many ways the effort raised provocative questions about values, ethics, medical research, and the nature of science.

Even after completing the series, I kept following the story. I couldn't stop. The stakes felt too high, the issues too complex, and the story too interesting to move on. I got to know more about the daily lives of the participants, visiting the families in their homes, watching the disease progress in the children and the toll it took on them and their loved ones. Sadly, some of the children died while I was still writing this book.

I spent time with the scientists in their labs, trying to learn why it was so hard to be certain about results, and also getting to know them during the rare moments when they were not working. I was reminded that they too were parents. Most of all, I continued to grapple with the larger societal questions that the story raised—so much so that, to get a better purchase on them, I pursued a master's degree in bioethics at Harvard Medical School. In the years that followed, the story took promising and also devastating turns—and citizen science, as a movement, really took off. Journals and blogs devoted to the subject began to appear. It got easier for scientists and families to connect with and find one another. Parents of children with rare diseases and their allies—including parents who were part of the NPC disease collaboration—helped found an advocacy group called Global Genes, which offered support and advice on how to direct scientific research and sustain scientific collaborations in diseases that once languished from lack of resources and attention. Scientists and laypeople joined ranks to form a Citizen Science Association and started confronting some of the thorny ethical questions. The National Library of Medicine, which preserves important scientific publications, began collecting citizen scientists' blogs in order to include them in the official scientific record.

Given everything that was happening, I felt the only way to do the story justice was to write a book about it—this book. I did not intend to chronicle the history of NPC patient advocacy. I chose to highlight the views and perspectives of some, but not all, of the many players involved, gravitating toward those who not only propelled events in the narrative forward but also raised the most confounding questions along the way. The collaboration they all built helped change the way I think about science. The many achievements and setbacks they continue to experience is a reminder of how complex and important and difficult the whole process has been—and continues to be. It is a remarkable and inspiring story, despite the many difficulties.

Toward the end of the book-writing process, the Covid-19 pandemic erupted, overwhelming hospitals, shuttering schools, closing businesses, and killing millions of people around the world. Many of the issues that bedeviled the intimate collaboration between NPC parents and scientists were now being played out on a large, worldwide, public stage. In response to the Covid crisis, regulatory agencies made it easier for scientists to develop vaccines and therapies in record time. Journals allowed Covid-19 information to be freely and immediately shared online, available for study by scientists and citizen scientists alike. Patients, not professional scientists, were the first to notice that growing numbers of people still suffered debilitating and sometimes confounding symptoms months after they were infected with Covid-19. They even gave the disease its name, Long Covid.

This new group of citizen scientists started collecting data about themselves. They released patient-driven studies online—and found themselves cited as experts by the director of the NIH, who in a blog post about their work linked to their self-reported data alongside a paper published in a traditional scientific journal. The pandemic offers a historic opportunity to finally build an infrastructure that can both enable and grow citizen science. It is too soon to know if the sense of urgency and spirit of collaboration that marked the early days of Covid will continue once the acute phase of the pandemic starts to recede. I realize that there are scientists who likely still remain unconvinced that collaborating with citizen scientists is a good idea. They might continue to insist that only those with elite and specialized training can do the work they do, or raise concerns that people who are not professionals could end up pursuing questionable or even potentially dangerous treatments in a desperate attempt to save themselves or their loved ones. There are also certainly members of the public that don't see themselves as experts, capable of shaping and directing and participating in meaningful scientific research. Still, I like to think that after they read this book, they will be persuaded by the evidence and change their minds—just as the very best scientists often do.

WE THE SCIENTISTS

1

THE HERE AND NOW

Addison and Cassidy Hempel, identical twin girls, were born on January 23, 2004.

Their father liked to say that the girls had a birthday no one could forget. "Born on one, two, three, four," Hugh Hempel said.

In the hospital, for the first few days after they were born, the nurses called the girls Baby A and Baby B. Hugh and Chris, the twins' mother, had picked out three potential names if the children turned out to be boys: Clayton, Carson, and Cole. The names rolled off their tongues. But they couldn't agree on what to call the children if they turned out to be girls. They decided they wanted to see their faces first, and then decide.

The twins were supposed to be born at the Washoe Medical Center in downtown Reno, a short drive from the couple's home in a grassy enclave that boasted its own private golf course. But the evening Chris went into labor, the neonatal intensive care unit at the hospital was full with premature babies, so they got sent to another hospital a few miles away. By the time they arrived, it was 10:00 p.m. Chris had already been in labor for hours. The hospital scrambled to get a team together and rushed Chris into surgery for a caesarean section. By 11:15 p.m., the girls were born, arriving a minute apart. They each weighed less than five pounds. Their eyes were a dark blue that started to lighten as the days went on. They had clear skin, tiny button noses, and, in notes Chris made in their baby books, "inner ears shaped like hearts," along with mouths that reminded her of tiny rosebuds.

The couple requested that a whiteboard be brought into Chris's hospital room. Bleary from lack of sleep, they made a list of girls' names they both liked. Aileen, Annabel, and Annalis went up on the board. So did Addison and Cassidy. They decided on the last two because the names sounded melodious together; they were a pair, their fates intertwined. Hugh was the one who decided on the nicknames Addi and Cassi—spelled with no "e" at the end, he insisted. Cassi had a small birthmark on the left cheek of her bottom; the distinguishing mark allowed the new parents to tell the children apart.

Back at home, the twins shared a crib in a yellow nursery for the first month and a half and often slept cuddled next to each other. The sheets had stars and moons on them. Hugh put together all the furniture in the room himself. Both girls loved to stare at the spotted ladybug book their aunt bought them, and the colorful mobiles above the crib.

As time went on, the girls reached all their developmental milestones, often around the same time. They both rolled over on the bed at three months old, on the same night and at the same time, right before their evening bath. Addi learned to stick out her tongue, and Cassi quickly followed. At eight months, Cassi sat up for the first time. A week later, Addi did too.

The twins mimicked Chris when she made faces. The girls squealed in delight when Chris opened her mouth as wide as it could go or stuck her thumbs in her ears, waggling her fingers. Friends told Chris to cut her long black hair after the babies were born, but she loved the feel of the girls' fingers, tugging at her to come closer. The children pulled her into their orbit.

In the notes Chris kept of that hazy period, during days and nights filled with constant diaper changes and bottles and interrupted sleep, she tried to jot down the small details. She didn't want to forget a thing—how Addi wrinkled her nose when she smiled and the delight Cassi expressed when she screamed into the telephone. The girls loved to crawl on their father like he was a jungle gym. Hugh stood six foot five inches, and he let them clamber from his lap up his arms and shoulders. The girls were playful and engaged with each other.

After the girls were born, Chris's mother, Cathy, who lived nearby, came over frequently to help out with the round-the-clock diaper changes and feedings. Grandma Cathy was also a favorite babysitter. Chris and Hugh got to sneak away for a night out together to eat dinner and catch up or take a few hours away from the tumult at home to play a round of golf. Whenever Chris returned home, she found her mother cuddling with the girls in her arms. Grandma Cathy looked up in delight and always said the same thing about her granddaughters: "The girls are the cat's pajamas."

By December 2004, the girls were eleven months old. Cassi was able to take six steps and stand on her own. Addi also was standing and making a few tentative strides forward. They could climb stairs, hold sippy cups, and turn the cranks on the windows, sometimes so hard that the handles broke. Cassi clapped her hands when listening to music, and Addi raised her foot when dancing. By the age of two years, the girls had a whole list of words they could say; not just "Mama" and "Daddy" but also "money," "sippy," and "go." They loved to watch *Teletubbies* on television, and both recognized the In-N-Out burger sign with the distinctive yellow arrow, pointing it out to Hugh when he took them on long car rides to try to get them to take a nap.

Around the time of the girls' second birthday, Chris and the twins came down with the flu. Chris recalls never feeling so sick before in her life. The girls were vomiting and had difficulty eating or drinking. At the doctor's office, the pediatrician examined the twins and noted they both had enlarged spleens. She told Chris and Hugh it was probably nothing serious, but given how sick the children were, she wanted to run blood tests. To everyone's surprise, the girls were diagnosed with Epstein-Barr virus, or mononucleosis. The pediatrician told Chris that the large spleens were likely caused by the mono and would return to normal size after the infection got cleared from their bodies. She told Chris to bring the children in for a checkup once they felt better. A few months later, the girls appeared to be back to normal, but when they returned to the pediatrician's office, their spleens remained enlarged. The anomaly caught the pediatrician's attention. She suggested more tests.

This time, Chris and Hugh decided to take the girls to a genetics specialist at Stanford University for the blood tests and another physical exam. Chris made a notation of the event in the girls' baby books. There, amid the accretion of details describing a normal and happy childhood, the small and large milestones marking what until then had seemed like normal development, Chris recorded the first signs that something might be amiss. "You both contracted a terrible case of mononucleosis this year and we have been traveling to Stanford hospital to see special doctors," Chris wrote, adding, "You have been incredible angels through all the tests we have done."

THE DOCTORS AT STANFORD tested the girls' blood for various diseases, everything from cancer to immune disorders. They took X-rays and ran CAT scans. All the tests came back negative. The family went home. The doctors, Chris recalled, told her not to panic. The enlarged spleens were worrisome, but there were no other signs of a problem. The girls' development remained on a normal track. They did not seem to have any cognitive issues. Despite the doctors' reassurance, "I was panicking," Chris said, a low hum of anxiety she felt coursing throughout her body.

Chris started noticing other signs that something might be wrong. When the girls ran, their movements were stilted. They tottered along as if they might fall. At home, the girls occasionally held onto the walls for support when they walked. Their heads wobbled a bit, but the movement was subtle and when Chris tried to call Hugh's attention to it, he didn't detect a difference. Hugh described the girls as "big, lanky kids" and thought their size was the most plausible explanation for the lack of coordination.

"I'll admit Chris's instincts that something was wrong kicked in way before mine," Hugh said.

Chris's father, Jim, spent hours trying to teach the girls to ride their tricycles, but the twins never caught on. No matter how often he cheered for them, cajoled them, or encouraged them, the girls sat there, propped on the seats like dolls, their legs dangling, unable to figure out how to make the motion to advance the pedals. In the end, Jim and Chris often ended up pushing the girls themselves on the trikes, exploring the neighborhood.

Then, nine months after the bout with mono, the girls got very sick again. They ended up spending three days in the hospital with vomiting and high fevers. The girls still had enlarged spleens, and ultrasounds revealed enlarged livers as well.

An enlarged spleen and liver are typical symptoms associated with lysosomal storage diseases, an umbrella group of over fifty genetic conditions. The lysosome acts as the garbage disposal and recycling system of the cell. When proteins accumulate, the lysosome breaks them down, releasing them back into the cell in pieces so they can be used again. When something goes awry and the system doesn't function properly, toxins build up, causing problems that can range from seizures to cognitive deficits. Sometimes, the malfunction can be mitigated. Gaucher disease, for example, cannot be cured but has treatments that address the symptoms. Other lysosomal storage diseases, such as Tay-Sachs, lead to a child's inexorable decline and death.

Addi's and Cassi's blood were sent off to a lab that specialized in testing for most, but not all, of these disorders. Chris and Hugh anxiously awaited the results. The tests came back negative, but that did not quell Chris's mounting fears. Now she was certain something was wrong, and the doctors hadn't yet found it.

Chris was writing less in the girls' baby books during 2006 and 2007, increasingly preoccupied by her mounting concerns about the girls. There were still moments when the children seemed like ordinary, mischievous toddlers. Addi turned on all the water in the tub and filled it up, flooding the master bathroom. She drew all over the bathroom cabinet with Chris's new lipstick and dumped peanuts on her parents' bed. Cassi got a new pack of crayons and used them to draw on the freshly painted walls of the house.

But the girls' pediatrician suggested that Chris take the girls into the local hospital in Reno to be seen again by specialists. A pediatric oncologist from San Francisco ran a clinic at the Reno hospital every month. Maybe a fresh set of eyes on the girls' case would yield something new, the pediatrician suggested.

During the physical exam, the oncologist noted the girls tired easily when she asked them to do something. They didn't engage the way normal three-year-olds did. Chris and Hugh recounted how the girls frequently tripped on their toys, not noticing them on the floor. When the doctor reviewed the list of genetic tests that had already been performed, she realized that the girls had been tested for better-known lysosomal storage diseases like Gaucher and Tay-Sachs, but no one had tested the twins for Niemann-Pick disease type C. Unlike other lysosomal storage disorders, NPC disease could not at that time be confirmed with a blood draw and, as a result, was often an afterthought by doctors who suspected a genetic cause for a patient's symptoms. To test for NPC, doctors used a special device that punched a small hole in the patient's skin, performing a skin biopsy. Tissue cells were extracted and grown in a lab for several months in order to determine if cholesterol was getting stuck inside the lysosome. Only then was a diagnosis made. The girls underwent skin biopsies.

When Chris realized they would not learn the results for months, "I was screaming in the house. Three months? I was ranting and raving around here." As soon as the doctor raised the possibility of NPC disease, Chris looked it up on the internet. She learned the disease was fatal. She also discovered that what she had been observing for months, the girls' clumsiness, listlessness, and enlarged spleen and liver, were all symptoms of the disorder. The constellation of disquieting observations now made sense.

Chris didn't want to wait around for the test results. She went online and searched for a leading expert in NPC disease. NPC was extremely rare. Most doctors never saw a single patient their entire career, even at leading academic centers, which was another reason why the disease was often missed and took so long to diagnose. Chris's internet research landed on the name Marc Patterson at the Mayo Clinic in Rochester, Minnesota. Marc, a pediatric neurologist, was an expert in lysosomal storage disorders, and one of his main areas of research was NPC disease. As a younger doctor on a fellowship at the National Institutes of Health, Marc helped run some early clinical trials testing drugs to treat NPC. None worked; children continued to progress and die. After so many years treating patients, he figured he had diagnosed or at least seen at one time nearly every known person living with NPC in the United States, and many others around the world. Chris emailed the neurologist directly, begging for an appointment as soon as possible. Within a week, she and Hugh and the girls were on an airplane flying to Minneapolis. They rented a car and drove the rest of the way to Rochester.

Inside Marc's office, the girls clutched their favorite stuffed animals, matching mini golden retrievers, both named Maxi. Marc held up a finger in front of the girls' faces and instructed them to follow the finger with their eyes as he moved it up and down. Right away he noted that neither girl could gaze downward without moving her head, a hallmark of NPC disease. When the exam was over, the family sat on the couch. Marc broke the news to Chris and Hugh. In his expert opinion, the doctor told them, the girls had NPC disease. There was no cure. Most children diagnosed in early childhood like Addi and Cassi did not live past their teens.

Later, once they were back at home in Reno, Chris cried uncontrollably for days thinking about the girls' future, often to the point she could not catch her breath. But that afternoon in the doctor's office, sitting on the sofa, the girls playing with their toys like they did on any other ordinary day, Chris stayed focused on the here and now. She asked the doctor if there were any drugs that might slow down the disease's progression.

Many patients with the disease took a drug called miglustat, or Zavesca, the neurologist told them. The drug had been approved by the FDA four years earlier, in 2003, but for treating people with Gaucher disease, a different lysosomal storage disorder. A clinical trial run by Marc under the auspices of Actelion, the drug's maker, was underway with NPC patients, but formal market approval from the

FDA might still take years. In the meantime, because the drug was already approved for another disease, Marc was able to write a prescription for both girls.

The couple asked the doctor about what other drugs might be in the pipeline. He listed off others under consideration, including some with promising data in animals. Setting up and running clinical trials took years and enormous funding, Marc added. Given the realities of drug development, Chris recalled, "The doctor didn't think there was really anything that could be ready in time to save the girls' lives."

UNTIL THE GIRLS' DIAGNOSIS, Chris never gave much thought to science. Growing up in a small town outside San Francisco called Millbrae, the main focus of Chris's life was the basketball court. Her parents split up when she was seven years old. In the first years after her parents' divorce, Chris lived with her mother during the week and saw her father on weekends. By high school, Chris was a star basketball player, known for her ability to shoot under pressure. She traveled constantly for games, attracting the attention of college recruiters. Chris's mother remarried and decided to move farther away from Chris's school, so Chris moved in full-time with her father. He let her practice shooting hoops outside until late at night. He also didn't mind when she kept up the practice inside the house, throwing the basketball against the wall of her room while she lay in bed. He attended all her games, a quiet and regular presence in the stands. Chris played point guard, serving as the shot caller on the floor. Her team won championships, and Chris broke state shooting records. Competitive athletics, Chris said, taught her how to shut out any outside distractions. In a noisy gym filled with screaming spectators, Chris tuned out the noise, drove to the basket, and focused on sinking her shot.

Chris got a basketball scholarship to the University of California, Berkeley, and majored in political science. "I probably wouldn't have been able to go to college otherwise," Chris said. "My parents were just scraping by." After graduation, she gravitated toward public relations. One of her first assignments changed her life. She spent the day following a software executive around at a convention, where he demonstrated how fans of the 1994 World Cup soccer games could get scores live using a new web browser developed by a start-up company called Netscape. It was Chris's first close-up look at the internet, and she was hooked. She immediately sent her résumé to Netscape and soon got hired as employee number 132.

There were only three people working in the company's public relations department at the time, all young women, and they earned the nickname "the hens." Their job wasn't simply to sell a web browser; they were promoting a cultural revolution. They got one of the company founders on the cover of *Time*, photographed in his bare feet, hardly the traditional portrait of a nascent business titan. They talked about the internet in almost religious tones. The internet gave anyone access to information they wanted, leveling the playing field between experts and amateurs. People could immerse themselves in a new topic that interested them, identify others around the world with similar passions or concerns, and use email to instantly communicate with friends and colleagues at any time of the day or night.

The hens worked crazy hours, with little separation between work and regular life. Chris fueled herself with a stash of PowerBars she kept in a box underneath her desk. After a long day, people headed out together for drinks, frequenting a popular gathering spot in Palo Alto called the Empire Grill and Tap Room. On weekends, Chris organized runs around the Dish, a trail near Stanford University. People brought along bottles of wine and held picnics at the top, enjoying the spectacular view of the valley below. Or they'd drive out to Marin County, north of San Francisco, for day trips, exploring the art galleries and eating in the seafood restaurants. On Chris's twenty-eighth birthday, she organized a group to join her in Yosemite for the weekend, where they climbed Half Dome, one of the park's most demanding hikes.

Chris met Hugh at Netscape. Hugh was a fellow believer in the mission, employee number 161, working in the marketing department. Hugh had grown up in Boulder, Colorado, playing ice hockey. He went east for college, playing one year on the University of Vermont hockey team. He quit the team, frustrated that he wasn't given much ice time, and took a job as a bartender to pay for school. He too was excited by Silicon Valley and the promise of the internet. Hugh's first job had been in sales at IBM in New York. He moved out to California and joined Apple, "hawking Macs" for four years. He left the company in 1993 and spent a year building a house on Castro Street in San Francisco. Once it was done, he wanted to get back into the tech scene. His old boss from Apple joined Netscape and persuaded Hugh to come work for him there. It was Hugh's first experience at a start-up, and the pace amazed him. "People slept in their offices," Hugh said, "but it was so exciting. It didn't feel like work."

Chris and Hugh sometimes worked together on projects. Hugh was developing the company's website and giving a lot of interviews, and the two talked communications strategy. When they socialized, it was in a big group at work. One night, the head of the marketing department got a limo and invited everyone out to a party. "We all piled into this limo," Chris recalled. "I got scrunched up next to Hugh." She felt an instant connection with him, like an electric current running between them. At the party, they danced together then parted ways at the end of the evening, "but that was it," Chris said. "We knew we needed to be together."

At work, they kept things a secret for as long as they could. Then Hugh won a trip to Hawaii with other top performers on the sales team. Spouses and partners were invited to go, so Hugh asked Chris along. The first day of the trip, she showed up at the beach in a red bikini. "Everyone was looking at me saying, 'Why are you here?'" Chris recalled. From then on, they went public with their relationship. When they got married in 1999, their nuptials were featured in a business story about the growing trend of couples sending wedding invitations by email rather than regular mail.

By then, Netscape had been bought by AOL, and the couple was ready for something new. They cashed in their stock options and set out on a trip around the world, sending airline tickets to friends and family to join them at different stops in the twenty-two countries they visited along the way.

When they finally came home, the Hempels settled in Reno, Nevada. They made plans to build a house. If Hugh wanted to get back into the start-up scene, San Francisco was only a few hours' drive away. Chris figured she was done with that world. She knew exactly what she wanted to do next. "I wanted to be a soccer mom," she said.

CHRIS AND HUGH HANDLED the girls' diagnoses in different ways. Hugh realized the girls would eventually lose their ability to walk, so he started working outside with a crew to clear away the rocks and tree roots in the backyard. He installed a paved walkway made of pale slate stones that he made sure were smooth to the touch.

Chris retreated to the walk-in closet in her bedroom for hours every day, determined to learn everything she could about the disease that was killing her daughters. She rarely slept and often did not change her clothes. The suits and fancy outfits she used to wear for work hung in plastic bags, gathering dust. She sat on the floor in a bathrobe, searching the web for any information related to NPC disease.

Chris read stacks of papers published in scientific journals into the early hours of the morning, stopping only to catch a few hours of restless sleep. In a disease as rare as NPC, the field was small enough that she started to recognize many of the same scientists' names. Sometimes she emailed the authors, identifying herself as a parent of children with NPC disease eager to learn more about the condition. More often

17

than not, the scientists emailed back answers to her questions, willing to help educate someone whose children lived with the disease they studied in a lab.

At any hour of the day or night, she could communicate with families around the world just like her own. She joined an online chat group for parents of children with NPC disease, one of many patient communities springing up online that allowed people to connect and share their experiences. Parents organized bake sales, golf tournaments, and other fundraisers to support the work of two major patient advocacy groups, the National Niemann-Pick Disease Foundation and the Ara Parseghian Medical Research Fund, the latter group named for the famous coach of the University of Notre Dame football team who had three grandchildren with NPC disease. (All three children passed away before the Hempel children were diagnosed: Michael Parseghian in 1997, Christa in 2001, and Marcia in 2005.) The Parseghian foundation has raised over $45 million dollars for research. Both family-founded organizations contributed funds to a successful effort by NIH researchers in 1996 to identify the faulty gene that children inherited—one from each parent—in order to be born with NPC disease. Yet by the time Addi and Cassi were diagnosed in 2007, more than ten years since the identification of the gene had passed. Scientists still had not translated the important research discovery into an effective therapy for NPC disease.

Chris tapped into a stream of discontent that flowed through chat groups and patient sites and personal Facebook pages, expressing the same kind of frustration she felt over how science moved too slowly to keep up with the symptoms progressing in their loved ones. These patients felt science and scientists increasingly existed in a separate sphere from the public they were meant to serve. Some of the divide was due to the fact that modern research often addressed complex questions that required the use of specialized equipment in dedicated labs in order to run experiments. Science was a formal enterprise with regulations and infrastructure to go along with it.

These changes came with profound social consequences. Professionals gathered together in specialized conferences, talking almost exclusively to others sharing the same training, perspective, and approach to solving problems. A self-contained group of people reviewed and published one another's work in journals and essentially certified what counted as scientific knowledge.

Investigators were considered the experts, so they came up with the ideas about what experiments to run. They based their choices on all kinds of factors, not all of them scientific, such as personal interests, popularity in the professional world, and if funding was available. The questions they wanted to ask and hopefully answer were not always the ones that patients or their families considered the most crucial. Even if the academics' experiments generated important leads, drug companies often determined which moved forward because they held the purse strings to fund trials. The companies might select the drug they felt had the clearest path to regulatory approval. Or they might pursue the therapy that had the largest or most lucrative market. It was hard to recruit patients for clinical trials, and there were so many things that could go wrong, so companies sometimes steered away from diseases that seemed intractable or too uncommon.

Scientists at academic institutions did not typically receive grants to accelerate the development of drugs for those suffering right then. They worked mainly on basic research, questions aimed at gaining better understanding of the mechanisms of the disease. There was no real deadline for such exploration. Any insights regarding drug development that might emerge were more likely to help patients in the future than patients struggling at the moment.

Chris realized right away she was not the only one looking for a different approach. Some patients expressed their willingness to try any promising drug, even before it had been fully vetted in clinical trials with large numbers of patients. Others shared detailed logs and charts tracking their daily experiences, ideas for experiments, and theories about how to mitigate the symptoms of their disease. Chris was looking for a novel partnership, and amid the detritus of her old life, she turned up a promising lead. A group of parents whose children had NPC disease were gathering with scientists at the National Institutes of Health Chemical Genomics Center in Rockville, Maryland. The families and the scientists wanted to find a drug to treat NPC disease. To do it, they agreed to pursue science together. Three weeks after learning their children were going to die, the Hempels were on their way.

2

A DIFFERENT FEAR

n 1994, one-year-old Dana Marella served as a flower girl at her aunt's wedding. Dana had recently started walking and was a little clumsy going down the aisle. "We never thought anything of it," said her father, Phil. At least not at first.

A friend of Phil's parents, a doctor, attended the wedding and noticed Dana's awkward gait. Her right foot turned in a little. During the reception, amid the celebrating and cheers for the new couple, the friend was concerned enough that he took Phil aside and suggested that Dana go see a doctor. Soon after, Phil and Andrea, Dana's mother, took Dana to an orthopedist. The doctor found no structural abnormality in the little girl's legs or hips. "Everyone said she will grow out of it," Phil said.

Toward the end of kindergarten, Dana's teacher called the Marellas and asked them to come in for a meeting. "We love Dana," the teacher said. The little girl was vivacious, funny, and kind. She knew when a friend needed a hug. But Dana wasn't keeping up with the other kids in the classroom or at recess. She had trouble remembering things and slurred her words. At recess, she fell when she tried to run. The teacher's concern set off a search for a diagnosis that took Dana from doctor to doctor. Over the years, the folder with the test results grew thicker. The doctors agreed something was wrong, but no one knew what it was. They ran tests with inconclusive results and then sent the Marellas on to the next specialist. One preeminent neurologist, sitting in front of a wall full of testimonials from grateful patients and families, concluded Dana had permanent brain damage but no satisfying explanation for the cause. Other doctors examined Dana and admitted they were stumped. "It didn't make sense to us," Phil said. "She had been normal when she was born, and now she wasn't."

Finally, in 2001, after an appointment with yet another neurologist, the doctor directed the family to go see Marc Patterson. Marc saw the rarest of the rare diseases, the neurologist said. At the time, Dana was eight years old and her parents had been searching for a diagnosis for three years. "Marc knew in five minutes it was NPC," Phil said.

The couple was devastated to learn there was no cure for NPC, but Marc told them he and other investigators were working with a company to launch a clinical trial to test the drug Zavesca, which had showed promising results in mice with NPC. Marc anticipated a trial in NPC patients would launch soon; the Marellas hoped Dana could be part of it, and that the drug might stop the relentless progression of the disease.

With no other therapeutic options on the horizon, the couple returned to the large Greenwich, Connecticut, home they shared with Dana and her three siblings and tried as best they could to proceed with regular life. They attended church on Sundays, alternating between the traditional Catholic mass familiar from their own childhoods and a more modern ecumenical service filled with raucous music and Christian-themed songs that brought everybody to their feet in the auditorium of a local school. The Marellas felt supported by their communities, which rallied around Dana and the family. "Dana is a celebrity around here," Phil once told me. In church, Andrea sat in the back and quietly slipped outside with Dana if the girl had a seizure. On weekend afternoons, they liked taking their sailboat out on Long Island Sound. The children brought fishing rods and worms and sat on the boat, lines dangling, rarely catching any fish but enjoying the fresh air.

The couple felt frustrated that the timeline for the start of the Zavesca clinical trial kept slipping. The company developing the drug was small with limited resources; for business reasons, it pursued FDA approval first in Gaucher disease, a more common rare disease than NPC, which further delayed the start of an NPC trial. As time went on, Dana's symptoms got worse. She went from a walker to a wheelchair in order to get around. Phil and Andrea worried about her breathing and implemented a regimen of asthma medication, nebulizers, and regular physical therapy to try to keep the girl's lungs clear. The sailing outings continued, but Andrea held her daughter in her arms during the trips to ensure Dana didn't fall off the boat.

With four children in the house, there was always something to do. Julia, Dana's older sister, attended dance recitals; Philip, her older brother, played baseball; and Andrew, the baby of the family, trailed after them all, trying to keep up with his siblings. At the time of Dana's diagnosis, the three other children did not show neurological symptoms of NPC disease. Doctors advised them that it was their decision if they wanted to test the other children to see if they too had inherited the gene mutation for the disease. Since there were no effective treatments for the condition and the other children appeared healthy, the Marellas did not pursue genetic testing.

Then, in 2004, the Marellas got word that the Zavesca trial for NPC patients was finally getting started. They drove with Dana from Greenwich to the National Institutes of Health, where patients were tested to see if they qualified for enrollment in the clinical trial. Not all patients were guaranteed a spot. In order to determine if a new drug worked, investigators did not enroll patients with a disease that was too advanced. Even if a drug might have benefits, it might be impossible to detect any improvement in a seriously ill patient, the thinking went. When Dana completed the enrollment evaluation, doctors concluded the disease was now too advanced for her to participate in the trial. Phil and Andrea were devastated. They drove back home from the NIH in silence.

They wrestled again with the decision about whether to test their other three children to see if they also had NPC disease. Phil and Andrea still didn't notice any pronounced cognitive difficulties in the children, but they shared a sense of disquiet about Andrew, their youngest child. Like many people with NPC disease, Dana had an enlarged spleen, first picked up by a pediatrician during a routine childhood physical exam. Years before, Andrew's pediatrician had also noticed an enlarged spleen in the boy. "I think in our minds, we were afraid that whatever was wrong with Dana might also be wrong with Andrew, but we put the thought away," Phil said. They took Andrew for an examination with Marc. If Andrew did have the disease, they told Marc they wanted to enroll him in the Zavesca trial. "We decided we needed to know," Phil said.

After the exam, Marc concluded Andrew had NPC disease too, although the boy exhibited only mild symptoms. When Phil and Andrea inquired about enrolling their son in the Zavesca trial, they learned there were no more spots available. But because the drug was already FDA-approved for Gaucher disease, Marc was able to write prescriptions for both Dana and Andrew. The official clinical trial for Zavesca got underway. In Greenwich, Dana and Andrew formed a small Zavesca study of their own.

AFTER DANA'S DIAGNOSIS, the Marellas started a foundation called Dana's Angels Research Trust, or DART, to raise money for NPC research. DART ran small events and walks that raised around $25,000 a year. Andrew's diagnosis made the family realize they needed to raise larger sums. With Andrew, there was still a chance to change the course of the disease's progression, but only if researchers focused on accelerating the development of drugs. At the annual family support conference run by the National Niemann-Pick Disease Foundation that Phil attended, Marc was often asked at the end to give a speech, a kind of state-of-the-field address that summarized the latest research and hit on a larger message to inspire the community. Phil was struck by Marc's exhortation that basic research was not enough. Understanding how the NPC protein functioned was important, but that was not the only question to ask; certainly, to the parents, not the main or most important question at all. Marc said even if the Zavesca clinical trial succeeded, the drug alone was not going to be enough to stop the children from dying. They should think about Zavesca not as a cure, but rather as the first drug in an eventual drug cocktail, similar to the way HIV/AIDS patients were treated. More drugs were needed, urgently, Marc told the group. "He implored the researchers," Phil said about the neurologist's speech. "He said there is amazing science, but the researchers need to step back periodically and say, 'Can I turn any of this research into something for the children? Can I give this drug to someone? Did I learn something that will result in a drug?'"

Phil felt scientists would never ask those questions without a firm push; they had to be forced by the parents to take the step that Marc advised. "Ultimately what they love is to completely understand how cholesterol moves around the cell and gets processed," Phil said. The scientists who attended the annual scientific conferences and family meetings weren't, for the main part, drug developers; many of them weren't even clinicians who treated patients—they were lab scientists, at home amid test tubes and petri dishes. Phil wanted to do more than fund research into cholesterol. He wanted to fund drug development and experiments that might someday result in treatments for Dana and Andrew.

For their 2005 fundraiser, the Marellas decided to sponsor something splashier. Maybe they could even entice some celebrities to sign on. The couple often noticed television personalities Regis Philbin and his wife, Joy, who also owned a house in Greenwich, walking around town. One day, Andrea dropped off a letter at the Philbins' house, describing NPC disease and her dreams for her children's future and asking if they might consider attending the upcoming DART benefit. Andrea was shocked when the Philbins called and agreed to let the Marellas use their names on the DART posters going up all over town. "You write a powerful letter," Regis Philbin told Andrea.

But the Marellas didn't have a host for the evening. "I was thinking it might have to be me," Phil said. One evening, a week before the fundraiser, a woman who ran a store in town called Phil and told him that Frank Gifford, the former football player and sports announcer, had just been in the store and saw a DART poster hanging up. Frank and his wife, Kathie Lee, lived in town too and wanted to help. They were friends with the Philbins and also had a daughter the same age as Dana Marella. Phil called the Giffords and soon learned that the couple was willing to serve as the fundraiser's hosts. The Giffords even donated a prize for the event auction, an offer of dinner at their house for ten people. The dinner party was sold for $25,000. By the end of the evening, DART raised $250,000. Phil and Andrea spoke with Marc about how to use it to speed up drug development and started funding a series of small experiments testing different compounds.

Phil learned about the meeting at the NIH in late 2007 from another parent who also planned to attend. He jumped at the chance to build a novel partnership between parents and scientists. Many of the researchers, such as Marc Patterson, were people Phil already knew. DART had funded some of the scientists' NPC research. But the NIH meeting marked the first time Phil met the Hempels. Phil considered all the parents members of a large family, bound together by their children's cruel diagnosis. But temperamentally, they were not alike. Phil came from a more reserved world than the rough-and-tumble, aggressive style of Silicon Valley in which Chris and Hugh felt at home. Phil studied accounting and business in college, then worked days while he went to law school at night. He eventually got a job as general counsel at a media company that got sold to Paramount. Even then, working mainly as a consultant and on DART projects, Phil retained some of the traits of a corporate man. He thought before he spoke. He read all the fine print in a contract. He wanted to speed up the development of new drugs, but he wasn't exactly looking to overthrow the entire system.

Dana Marella and Addi and Cassi Hempel exhibited a more progressed disease than many of the children of the other parents who initially joined the collaboration. The parents still sometimes found themselves on different sides of debates about how quickly to use experimental compounds in the children. But they shared common ground on one key aspect. Although all the parents lived with the fear their children were in imminent danger, one of the parents noted about the Marellas and the Hempels, "It's a different fear you live with."

3

THE FISHING EXPEDITION

Forbes D. Porter—or Denny, as everyone called him—knew from an early age that he wanted to be two things: a farmer and a doctor. He joined a Boy Scout troop in the first grade in the rural town outside Pittsburgh where he grew up. Over the years, he learned how to navigate through the woods, leaving a trail of small signs to help find his way back. He practiced building a campfire and quickly learned that the best place to pitch a tent is on flat ground, preferably with a cushion of pine needles or dirt underneath the sleeping bag. He could imitate a bird's whistle. Eventually, he became an Eagle Scout.

He studied science and medicine at Washington University in St. Louis, until then the farthest he had ever traveled from home, and took odd jobs to help pay for school. The university promised to try to place students in part-time jobs relevant to their future careers. Denny put down medicine on the form, hoping to get work in a lab. Instead, he got assigned to wash dishes in one of the kitchens at a campus dining hall. He stuck it out for a week, then wrote a letter to the head of the program, explaining that he was hoping for work more related to the medical profession. This time, he got assigned to the archaeology lab. The lab was tucked away in a basement. The light was dim; there was a constant hum of generators. The lab director was back from a dig and needed help sifting through bins of dirt, separating important bits of the past like fossils and bones from the rocks. Denny didn't mind the job. He liked to watch the small pile of bones grow higher.

Denny's original plan was to go to medical school and then work as a doctor in a rural area. But he felt intrigued by research and genetics and decided to stay in St. Louis to get a PhD as well as a medical degree. During his genetics fellowship, he was moonlighting in the emergency room of the local hospital to earn extra money. One Friday evening, soon after arriving home from a long shift, he got a call for a genetics consultation on a newborn baby. Genetics consultations weren't usually considered emergencies and no one asked him to turn around and come immediately back in, but the child's case fascinated him. Denny didn't want to wait another moment. He headed back to the hospital that same night in order to see the child.

He found the baby wrapped in a blanket in an incubator in the neonatal intensive care unit. Even late at night, the unit hummed with the sound of monitors and alarms. Nurses scurried to attend to crying children. Denny held the baby in his arms, studying him with a mix of detachment and wonder. The child had a serious heart defect that was going to need repair, fused second and third toes, and a cleft palate. None of the doctors knew exactly what the child had. They suspected a genetic condition, probably something rare since they weren't sure what the various symptoms might mean.

To Denny, the baby's problems presented a puzzle that he wanted to solve. Even as a young doctor, Denny knew there weren't a lot of traditionally happy endings in genetics consultations. When the doctors called him in, it was usually because they had already run through the gamut of common problems that they recognized and could immediately fix with surgery or treat with medicine. Denny arrived on the scene when the doctors' suspicions steered toward something very bad; if not life-threatening, then definitely life-changing. When talking to parents, Denny saw his task as separating fact from opinion or speculation, and being clear when his own views differed from other ones that were also available. He talked in measured tones with a calm demeanor; his work, and his personality, gravitated toward solid ground.

That evening in the emergency room, Denny took note of each anomaly, small and large. Then he started looking through the computer databases for case reports. He was checking to determine if there were other babies whose medical histories might match the child in intensive care. He pored through textbooks, trying to piece together the available clues and fit them into a coherent narrative. At two o'clock in the morning, he believed that he had finally found the answer. He diagnosed the baby with a cholesterol metabolism disorder called Smith-Lemli-Opitz syndrome, or SLOS, a genetic condition where people don't make enough cholesterol. The condition caused a range of problems, from the mild to the very serious. The baby had a severe form, and Denny did not think he would live very long. He gave the doctors his report and went back home again to sleep. He never saw the baby again.

His stint in the emergency room came to an end soon afterward, and he moved to the Washington, DC, area to work in a genetics lab at the National Institutes of Health. But he never forgot the baby in the emergency room. When he was offered the chance to run a lab at the NIH and asked where he wanted to focus his research, he said SLOS.

Despite his passion for research, Denny didn't want to work only in the lab. He was also a practicing pediatrician, shuttling between the two worlds of lab research and clinical care, each of them informing his work in the other. He ran SLOS studies in the lab and also took care of children with the condition, getting to know their families. The parents were the ones who told Denny they had been giving their children a common dietary supplement to try to increase the children's cholesterol levels. The parents said the supplement seemed to work. The children's behavior was less aggressive and hyperactive. Denny and some other investigators decided to set up a clinical trial to test the idea.

The study required the children to stop taking the supplement for a two-week period. Denny estimated he needed forty children to enroll in order to gather enough data to tell whether the improvements the parents noted were due to the supplement or to chance. Only ten children enrolled.

"The parents were afraid to enroll the kids," Denny said. "They worried the children's behavior would go off the charts if they stopped. They wanted to know why we were running a trial at all since they were already sure it worked." Denny closed the trial without ever getting a definitive answer. In a paper Denny and his colleagues later published, they wrote that based on the small amount of data they managed to collect, they had seen no difference in hyperactive behavior when the children took the dietary supplement and when they did not, results that "call into question anecdotal reports" of benefits.

Denny's SLOS work attracted the notice of several NIH colleagues who were veterans in the NPC research world, including one who had been part of the team of researchers that successfully identified the gene defect that caused NPC disease. They knew he was interested in genetic problems involving cholesterol. They had one. At a recent NPC disease conference, a scientist presented results from testing a compound known as allopregnanolone in mice with Niemann-Pick disease type C. The NIH doctors were excited by the data. The mice were living for months when treated with the drug, more than double previous experiments done in the animals using other compounds. The results were preliminary, and the experiment needed to be replicated by other scientists. But at the NIH, the researchers felt the time had come to at least start thinking about how to eventually set up a clinical trial in children if the original findings held up. Denny had run the SLOS trial. They wanted him to consider doing the same in NPC disease.

The request launched Denny's entry into the NPC research world. Denny sat with the researchers as they walked him through the allopregnanolone results. Denny's first question was practical: How did they plan to measure whether the drug was working? In the mice, the scientists measured changes in the amount of cholesterol stored in the animals' neurons by killing the animals and then studying small slices of their brains. No one knew how to measure improvement in a child. Even after years of basic research, doctors still weren't sure exactly how the disease progressed. Each child seemed to present symptoms in a different way, at different ages. Patients declined at variable rates. Some children were more affected cognitively, slurring their words, unable to focus. Others exhibited a jerky gait and soon lost the ability to walk. Denny wasn't sure how to go about proving the drug worked in a trial in a way that the Food and Drug Administration would accept.

So Denny proposed that they first set up what was called a natural history study. A natural history study was very different from a clinical trial, which was designed to evaluate promising drugs. Scientists ran natural history studies as massive information-gathering operations, almost like a medical version of a fishing expedition. They wanted to understand how slowly or rapidly a disease progressed. They collected detailed information about the symptoms and how the disease damaged organs. The studies were often considered a first step in a process that might eventually lead to the launch of a clinical trial. The findings could help investigators identify symptoms that were most important to treat if they wanted to improve the patients' outcome. If a drug trial was eventually launched, data from the participants in the natural history study could sometimes serve as the comparison arm against which scientists measured outcomes in order to determine if an experimental compound was actually changing the course of the disease.

Denny wasn't initially sure how many people might agree to participate when he launched the natural history study in 2006. Enrollment required coming once a year for a week of testing at the NIH. Parents had to take time off from work. If they had other children, particularly those who were school age, they had to make arrangements for childcare. Denny set a modest goal of recruiting twenty-five people. He eventually ended up with 138 participants. He was moved by the enthusiasm and commitment of the parents who started arriving at the NIH from all over the country, children in tow. Denny tried to gather data on everything—the children's height and weight, how they walked, talked, listened, and swallowed. He took blood and urine; he performed lumbar punctures to obtain cerebral spinal fluid.

Denny's office started to fill with small offerings, tokens of affection for the doctor trying to shine a light on a very rare disease—colorful drawings, a dangling Santa Claus doctor figurine, a wooden plaque with a small red ball poking out of the middle.

Denny had a view from his office of a small patch of

grass where the children in the natural history study some-times gathered to get fresh air when they were in between tests. The parents brought plastic bats, balls, and mitts with them to keep the children entertained. Sometimes, when Denny had time, he joined them, squatting down on the ground to catch or taking a turn pitching the ball right over the plate, then pretending to be an announcer calling out in excitement as children rounded the makeshift bases.

WHEN CHRIS AUSTIN, the head of the NIH's Chemical Genomics Center, opened up his lab in November 2007 for a meeting between parents of children with NPC and scientists, Denny wasn't surprised to be on the guest list. In a short period of time, he had turned himself into a leading expert on NPC disease. He knew some of the families who planned to attend the meeting. Phil Marella's children had been among the first to enroll when Denny opened the natural history study.

In contrast to some of the parents and scientists going to the meeting, however, Denny wasn't searching for a new model for science. He knew the scientific process did not move quickly enough for the children in his care, but he believed in the rigor of the scientific process. He was skeptical of finding shortcuts when it came to developing drugs. It took time to unravel the scientific underpinnings of poorly understood diseases. If scientists and parents moved too quickly, they could end up with a situation similar to his SLOS trial—trying remedies they believed were beneficial but likely did not work.

Nonetheless, despite any reservations he might harbor about how quickly scientists could find an effective drug, Denny recognized that his research could benefit from and contribute to the collaborative. The NIH's genomics center offered access to advanced technology such as robots that could test more promising drugs in a week than Denny could likely accomplish in years in his own lab. The opportunity to generate new leads for drugs that might help children with NPC disease was not something Denny could pass up. If all went well, Denny planned to propose at the meeting that Chris Austin's team work with him to run experiments testing drugs on skin cells that Denny collected from the children in the natural history study.

Denny was an avid fisherman in his free time. His grandfather had owned acres of land containing black cherry trees. When Denny and his cousins sold some of the trees to lumber firms, Denny used a portion of the proceeds to buy an eighteen-foot fishing boat that he named the *Serotina*—the scientific name for the trees.

Denny tried to arrange his work schedule during trophy rock fishing season in the spring so he could take the boat out early on the Chesapeake Bay. He always stopped to talk to the old-timers sitting on the dock before he cast off, hoping to glean a few tips on where the fishing was good that day. He cut up the worms for bait and filleted the fish right on the boat, throwing the guts and carcasses back into the bay.

Most times, the bay felt like a large basin, waves sloshing from side to side. But in bad weather, it could be difficult to navigate the choppy waters. Denny had been caught when a storm came out of nowhere, the waves surging. Grabbing the sides of the boat to hold himself steady, he listened to the pop and ting of screws giving way and falling to the boat floor. The pounding of the waves reverberated through every bone. The only thing to do when that happened, he said, was stand up straight, brace himself, and try to find a way back.

Out on the water, boaters were part of a community. If they raced their boats too fast, the waves created in their wake could swamp another boat. They needed to pay attention to where others were going. The rules about how to act on the water weren't written down, Denny said, but derived from shared customs and expectations. Denny had decided long ago that in both fishing and science, he was willing to drop a few lines off the back of the boat and wait patiently to see if there were any bites.

4

THE CATALYSTS

Marc Patterson had traveled all over the world taking care of NPC patients. He went to Argentina at the behest of a family that needed an expert to figure out a treatment strategy for their child. He attended meetings sponsored by families of NPC patients in Germany, Spain, and England, forging relationships that spanned decades. But in April 2007, he embarked on a journey to Brazil that was unlike anything he had ever done before.

Marc—along with two other NPC scientists and the parent of a child with the disease—had been invited to stay at the home of Luiz Cezar Fernandes, a Brazilian businessman whose daughter, Renate, had been diagnosed with NPC disease in 1992 when she was in her early twenties. Now Renate was thirty-eight years old, an age that not many patients with NPC disease ever reached. In the early years after the diagnosis, Renate's family sought help from leading genetic disease experts all over the world. They brought Renate to meet doctors and researchers in New York City and Lyon, France. Everywhere they went, they heard the same thing. There was no effective drug to treat NPC, no available therapy that could stop the disease.

So the family decided to create their own treatment plan with the aim of extending Renate's life for as long as possible. They lived on a large, well-secured estate in Petrópolis, a mountainous city about a ninety-minute drive from Rio de Janeiro. Petrópolis had once been the imperial seat of Brazilian kings. Wealthy and prominent Brazilian families built homes there to escape the heat. Within the Fernandes compound, the family assembled a diverse team of healthcare providers. The group included a geneticist and metabolic specialist, as well as an orthopedist, neurologist, pharmacologist, lung physiotherapist, and audiologist. There were piano and singing instructors—Renate loved music—and an art therapist. Every two months, everyone assembled in the large dining room, which had doors that opened onto the veranda and offered a stunning view of the rain forest. Everyone from the art therapist to the geneticist assessed Renate's progress and made suggestions for any necessary changes. They worked together to create a flourishing and dynamic medical ecosystem, with Renate's needs at the center of all they did. The model the Fernandes family had come up with was designed to promote longevity in a disease for which there was still no effective drug.

For Marc, the journey to Petrópolis represented a change in the traditional role he usually played. Marc had been born and educated in Australia before arriving in 1988 at the Mayo Clinic in Rochester, Minnesota, expecting to stay for a one-year fellowship. He extended for a second year. When the time was up, he got offered the chance to join the staff. Despite the harsh winters, he agreed, but he first took a detour for more specialized training in metabolic diseases at the National Institutes of Health in Bethesda, Maryland. At the NIH, Marc joined the lab of Roscoe Brady, a renowned scientist in the field of lysosomal storage disorders. Roscoe's lab discovered that individuals with Gaucher disease, the most common lysosomal storage disorder, lack a crucial enzyme. It took decades of additional work but Roscoe's team built on that finding to help develop an effective enzyme replacement drug to treat Gaucher patients. Members of Roscoe's lab also led a team that identified the specific gene defect that caused the majority of cases of Niemann-Pick disease type C. Yet unlike in the case of Gaucher disease, despite the advances in basic science, NPC therapies remained elusive.

. . .

DURING HIS NIH FELLOWSHIP, Marc spearheaded a clinical trial testing statins in NPC patients, one of the early attempts to treat NPC disease with a system-wide intervention rather than addressing individual symptoms as they emerged. The scientists hypothesized that the large amount of unprocessed cholesterol stuck in the cells might be reduced through the combination of a low-cholesterol diet and a regimen of cholesterol-lowering drugs. They enrolled twenty-five patients, taking liver biopsies before the patients were treated to try to measure how much cholesterol was in the tissues, and then again after four months on the therapy.

The trial failed. The patients' blood cholesterol levels dropped, but the diet and the drugs did nothing to stop the neuron damage that was one of the most insidious aspects of the disease. When the fellowship ended and Marc returned to the Mayo Clinic, he figured he had left the lab behind. He wanted to focus full-time on caring for patients. But as one of the foremost experts in an extraordinarily rare genetic disease, Marc was sought out for advice not only by families but also by potential drug developers. He agreed to help design and run a clinical trial of Zavesca for the company Actelion. The company was trying to determine if the medication, a pill that had been approved by the FDA for Gaucher patients unable to take enzyme replacement therapy, might also benefit people with NPC disease. Even though Marc believed Zavesca helped ameliorate some of the disease's symptoms, he knew it was not a cure. NPC remained a fatal disease.

Over the years, Marc had come to believe that scientists needed a new approach if they were going to find a cure. The traditional scientific model, the very one in which Marc had been trained, relied on scientists working at lab benches, conducting experiments under the demanding oversight of charismatic senior scientists. The main ways of communicating discoveries to the wider community were through the publication of papers (a laborious process that could take months, if not years) or the sharing of selected, partial information with other scientists via presentations at annual professional conferences. The system was cumbersome and slow. It might work for basic research, generating over time more leads and additional knowledge, but, Marc acknowledged, the approach had not successfully moved the needle on keeping NPC patients alive. Doctors like Marc were no closer to having a cure, a situation that he wanted to help change. But where he got stuck was in trying to come up with an alternative model that he could trust to more rapidly develop safe and effective drugs.

In the months leading up to the Brazil trip, Marc and his companions had started talking about what needed to change. They decided to write down their ideas, and emailed the document, a work in progress, back and forth. They had no idea what might become of their vision; it was still inchoate. But what was already clear to Marc was that changes were happening. After all, Marc had always been the expert, invited all over the world to impart knowledge. Now he was going to Brazil to gain it.

THE FOUR MEN ARRIVED in Rio on a Friday and were met at the airport by a driver and one of the scientists working with the Fernandes family. Petrópolis, a city of around 250,000 people, sat eight hundred meters above sea level. Marc could feel the change in the climate as the car wound its way around the turns in the narrow roads. The family home was located on a secluded estate that also functioned as a working sheep ranch. The big double doors at the entrance shut behind them. They didn't leave the compound for the next four days.

After arriving, they sat on the patio and took in the stunning views. Luiz's wife, Cecelia, greeted them. Renate sat in a wheelchair, dressed to meet the guests. Her fingernails were painted and her eyes were expressive. She had suffered a bad case of pneumonia the year before, landing her in the hospital intensive care unit for seventy-two days and requiring a tracheotomy. They had been sitting there only a short while when Luiz joined them, bringing out a bowl of freshly baked cheese puffs.

There was no formal schedule over the next days of their visit. They were staying in a luxurious pool house. The men woke early to the sounds of toucans outside. Marc swam laps for thirty minutes every morning in the pool. There were two sit-down meals each day in the dining room where the Fernandes family and their guests gathered together, discussing world politics, the global economy, and the culture of Brazil. They took long, leisurely walks together around the compound. They visited with Renate and listened with her to music; she loved disco music and was a fan of the Bee Gees and the song "Stayin' Alive." One afternoon, Luiz drove them around the estate on his Land Rover. "It felt like we were in Shangri-la," said Daniel Ory, one of the NPC scientists on the trip. Far away from their daily responsibilities, ensconced in the verdant setting, the men engaged in freewheeling discussions about how to develop a new model for science.

Marc and his three companions were not alone in thinking about ways to spark more effective collaboration in science. The National Science Foundation, which provided funding for many grants, had issued new scoring guidelines requiring scientists to discuss in their proposals how they were going to work together. A Michigan scientist had proposed forming what he called "collaboratories," using technology to enable labs around the world to share data and work on joint projects. Most of these early initiatives, however, assumed that the central problem was that scientists did not talk to one another or share data. As a result, the proposed solutions focused on ways to promote more real-time interactions through the use of video chatting or the creation of wikis and other types of online platforms where scientists could share data and solicit the insights of their colleagues.

Before the trip, the proposal Marc and the others came up with followed a similar trajectory, offering suggestions about recruiting labs with different specialties, dividing up tasks, sharing information openly and frequently, and working together toward the primary goal of drug development. Perhaps Luiz Fernandes might invest in the concept, they speculated, give them some seed money to create a pilot project. Marc even came up with the name for the proposed collaboration: Support of Accelerated Research for Niemann-Pick C, or SOAR.

But there in Petrópolis, the problem could be viewed in a different way. The obstacle wasn't only that scientists didn't collaborate with one another. It was also that scientists didn't collaborate with patients and families—certainly not in the intimate, intense, and egalitarian way that they were witnessing. Renate was not just a body to be studied; she was the hub of a vast universe, encompassing her family and the community in which they lived. The luxurious amenities Renate's family provided were unavailable to most people, but surely the underlying approach was worth analyzing. The system the family created generated data from every aspect of Renate's life and focused relentlessly, single-mindedly, on how to address the challenges of a patient with the disease. All ideas were welcome. The art therapist had a seat at the table, as did the occupational therapist and the neurologist and the parents and the patient herself.

In thinking about how to apply the model, there were many elements to work out. It wasn't clear if scientists would agree to participate. The precise role of patients and families and their potential contributions was not well-defined. "I don't think we fully understood what might happen if what the parents had in mind and what the scientists had in mind turned out to be rather different," Daniel said.

At the end of the trip, they gathered again in the dining area and made a presentation to Luiz. They discussed the lack of collaboration among scientists and its relation to the failure so far to find an effective drug to treat NPC disease. They suggested the initial components of a research alliance that they hoped could produce better results. Luiz listened attentively and asked questions, but Marc and the others did not get the sense he was going to invest in the pursuit of a new model. Even so, the four men left Brazil with the feeling the trip had been a tremendous success. They had new ideas, a foundation upon which to build. And when the four of them attended the meeting in Chris Austin's lab seven months later, the experiences in Petrópolis were catalysts for the ideas discussed that day. It was too soon to tell if a system like the one the Fernandes family had built could be replicated outside the walls of Petrópolis, but by the time he left Brazil, Marc knew he wanted to give it a try.

5

THE OPERA SINGER

Chris Austin was the neurology resident on call one evening in 1989 when a severely ill patient arrived by ambulance to his hospital in Boston. The patient had late-stage amyotrophic lateral sclerosis, or ALS, a fatal neurological disorder also known as Lou Gehrig's disease, that paralyzed people's muscles. The man had signed a do-not-resuscitate order and wanted to die at home, but because of a mix-up, the paramedics revived him. Angry that his wishes had been disobeyed, the man requested that the ventilator keeping him alive be shut off. Doctors at the hospital complied with the patient's plea. The twenty-nine-year-old Chris sat with the family at the bedside, watching as a life ebbed away. It took three hours before the man took his final breath.

Through the long and agonizing vigil, Chris felt increasingly enraged not only at his own helplessness but at a system that seemed to be failing its most central task: healing the sick. Chris had undergone years of grueling and intense training at some of the top institutions in the country. He graduated summa cum laude in biology at Princeton University, earned his medical degree from Harvard Medical School, and was accepted for a top-tier neurology residency at Massachusetts General Hospital, one of the premier hospitals in the country. He was the product of the best that medicine had to offer, and yet in his retelling of the story, he couldn't offer much. He always emphasized that his job that evening was to "turn off the monitors when the patient died." His moral distress that he could not do more shook him to the core.

"I loved neurology," Chris said. He also recognized the real value a doctor could provide by offering comfort and advice and care even when a cure was not available. "Sick patients need doctors to take care of them," he said. "While we may not have the greatest treatments, the patients still need us to be with them on this journey and do what we can, and that's a really important function."

The diseases Chris encountered most frequently in the neurology clinic were intractable and devastating. Huntington's disease relentlessly destroyed nerve cells in the brain. Alzheimer's disease stripped people of their memories and identity. Chris's patients came into the office seeking hope and, more often than not, he had no effective therapy to offer. He usually wasn't even able to point to a promising drug on the horizon. "I couldn't stand simply telling patients with incurable neurological diseases that there was nothing we could do for them and having that be my life's work," Chris recounted.

As a doctor, Chris saw one patient at a time and tried to alleviate their symptoms. He valued the relationships he developed with his patients and their families. Working in a neurology clinic, taking care of people over the course of many years, gave him insight into the magnitude and burden of the diseases he treated. He saw the devastation that the loss of memory, abilities, and function wreaked, not only on the patient but also on loving family members, friends, and colleagues who struggled to help. The reverberations from the death of a single person affected an entire community. Chris tried hard to improve patients' lives, but he decried the system that left him with so few options. He wanted to try to change the course of the disease not only for the person sitting in front of him but also for "the many, many patients out there, even those I won't see," he said.

He set out to understand the ecosystem of medicine. He joined the lab of Constance Cepko, a developmental biologist and geneticist at Harvard Medical School. He figured that by studying genetics, his findings might lead to advances in the field, potentially reaching more people than he could care for in a clinic. In the lab, he learned the foundations of basic genetics, devising experiments with model organisms such as mice and fruit flies that sometimes shared important common genes with humans. One of the first papers Chris coauthored after joining the lab was published in 1990 in the journal *Development*. For that paper, he dissected the brains of twelve mouse embryos in order to study the patterns of the cells as they migrated through the animals' developing cortexes. It was very far from what he had been doing as a doctor treating patients in a clinic, but he loved "the elegance of basic genetics and what we can discover in the lab."

While Chris spent most of his time running experiments in the lab, he continued to see neurology patients, moonlighting at Massachusetts General as well as at a community hospital that had a walk-in clinic where patients with no insurance could come in off the street. He also pursued his passion for music. All his life, he loved to sing. In college and medical school, he studied music and voice along with biology and science. He tried out for parts in operas—he was a bass baritone—and earned extra money performing in two to three a year. As a first-year medical school student, he got to sing Beethoven's *Fidelio* at Lincoln Center for the Performing Arts in New York City. He continued to take on a variety of roles even as his career as a doctor flourished. He performed the part of the Calvinist chaplain who tries to bring order in the midst of chaos in *Lucia di Lammermoor*. In another production, he sang an aria from Mozart's *The Marriage of Figaro*. Chris could feel the exhilaration of the audience responding to the words he sang.

Opera also reminded Chris of the harmony he often felt was missing in the practice of medicine. Music was about the whole person. An opera represented an entire ecosystem, encompassing diverse perspectives and often communicating a common truth that drew in the people who listened. Even amid the extravagant costumes, people could relate to the human emotion displayed onstage. The stories were situated in a world filled with knaves and heroes, deadbeats and those who rose above their station. Ordinary people rubbed elbows with the highborn and the noble. Chris wondered why science couldn't be more like opera, where everything and everyone was connected.

Science and the scientists who loved and practiced it were isolated from the people they wanted to help and needed to engage in order to advance. "Research is ultimately about the patient, about humanity," Chris said. "But on a day-to-day basis, it is divorced from that. Opera is all about the human crucible. What makes humans human, what makes them think, what makes them sick, what makes them well." Music offered a different way, he said, "to ask the same question that always interested me: What makes the human organism what it is?"

Everywhere he looked, he saw a divide. Researchers didn't focus on the body as a whole, but rather specialized in its many different parts; cancer doctors treated the breast, prostate, or brain as if they were separate entities, even though the gene mutations that caused cancer in one organ might be the same in another, or located along common molecular pathways. Drugs that were already being prescribed for one disease might be useful in treating another, but there was no systematic program that tried to identify these compounds. In Chris's own life, he saw a large gap between the results of his elegant genetics experiments in the lab and their lack of relevance when it came to treating or trying to improve the lives of the people who crowded into the clinic. He lived in two separate worlds that rarely communicated. "The wonders of what I was doing in the lab had truly nothing to do with and no impact on what I saw in the clinic," he said.

After six years in the genetics lab, Chris now had training in both the clinical and research sides of neurology but was no closer than before to finding a way to bridge the divide between them. "There has to be a place to pull both of these worlds together," he thought.

He decided to try the pharmaceutical industry next.

Drug companies in the 1990s were increasingly interested in trying to find a way to harness genetic data to develop better, more targeted therapies. Chris was in the lab in 1995 when the head of research at the pharmaceutical company Merck came to visit Harvard. The executive told the scientists that Merck was creating a new genetics research department and was recruiting. The drug company wanted to be on the forefront of a new era of more personalized medicine. Chris immediately applied.

He started working at Merck in 1996, convinced he had finally found the place to investigate his disparate interests. "I was the brain guy," Chris said. He was charged with finding new ways to intervene in the progression of diseases such as Alzheimer's and schizophrenia, conditions for which there was a desperate need for treatments. Genetic information might help pinpoint an Achilles' heel in a disease and lead to the development of a drug to treat what Chris called the "rogues' gallery" of conditions that still perplexed doctors and killed patients.

But soon after his arrival in West Point, Pennsylvania, where Merck's research lab was based, Chris discovered he didn't know as much as he thought about developing drugs. The biggest problem, he learned, was overcoming the obstacles that stood in the way of turning a great idea into an actual drug that could make a difference in people's lives.

There was a long period of time that stretched years and cost tens of millions of dollars between the discovery of a novel finding and the launch of clinical trials. Most drugs failed during that stretch, at such frequent rates that drug developers called it "the Valley of Death." Even when things seemed to be going well, something often occurred out of the blue to disrupt the progress. "It was where all predictability goes away," said Chris.

In the Valley of Death, promising ideas got dropped for any number of reasons. Perhaps the compound corrected the disease in cells but was a dud in mice. Or the drug dramatically slowed down the progression of the disease but had such toxic side effects that a human being could not tolerate it for long. Sometimes a drug appeared both safe and effective but metabolized so quickly in the body that the chemists estimated someone would have to swallow a pill every fifteen minutes in order to see any benefit. It was maddening how making a small change in the chemical structure of a drug affected so many other things, setting off a chain reaction the scientists could not always foresee or even control. So much about the interaction of genes within the body remained a mystery, no matter how hard they tried to penetrate the secrets. Chris said he knew people who had spent decades at Merck toiling on one drug or another and had never seen a single one make it the entire distance through clinical trials in humans and approval by the Food and Drug Administration. He started to wonder if he was going to be one of them.

Most drugs, probably over 90 percent, Chris estimated, failed for one reason or another, and when they did, the money invested was lost. Given the odds, Chris understood why it was hard to gain traction for many of his ideas, especially since his focus was the brain, an organ that was still not well understood and was protected by a formidable barrier of cells that made it hard for many molecules to reach it.

"You balance the risk with the return and organizations like pharma tend to be risk averse," Chris said. He spent years on one key project doing research about a novel Alzheimer's target called gamma-secretase, only to see the compounds Merck developed ultimately go nowhere because of the drugs' toxic side effects.

Companies also dropped drug programs for reasons that weren't scientific at all, but related to the vagaries of business. The internal champion of a particular drug might leave the company, taking any enthusiasm and commitment to seeing the project through with them. Or funding ran out more quickly than anticipated and the top executives decided that continuing the program was akin to throwing good money after bad. A company might get bought by new owners who wanted to focus on a different disease and shelved an existing drug program. Diseases with a small patient market size such as ALS had an even more difficult road. The risk of failure was often deemed too great, the amount of investment required too high, and the potential path to market approval by the FDA too uncertain for companies to want to try at all. All the problems that plagued drug development overall were even more formidable in very rare diseases.

After six years at Merck, Chris felt just as frustrated by the realities of drug development as he had working in the neurology clinic and the genetics lab. Earlier in his stint at Merck, Chris met Francis Collins, then the director of the National Human Genome Research Institute, part of the NIH. (Francis later served as the NIH director from 2009 to 2021.) Francis had given a talk at Merck about his work as one of the leaders of the Human Genome Project, the multibillion-dollar international research effort that sequenced the human genome. After years of effort and money, the researchers announced in 2000 that they had a rough draft of the human genome, an incredible feat of ingenuity and technology. Francis and other scientists were figuring out how to apply the new knowledge to drug development, and Chris wanted to be part of that effort. By November 2002, he was ensconced at the NIH as senior adviser for translational research to Francis.

Chris's new boss had an interest in rare diseases. In 1989, Francis helped identify the gene mutation that caused cystic fibrosis, a life-threatening inherited disease that caused severe damage to the lungs and other organs. He invited a physician, who was also the mother of a boy with the ultra-rare rapid aging disease Hutchinson-Gilford progeria, to work in his lab searching for the genetic mutation that led to the development of the disease. The mother was a coauthor of the scientific paper describing the result.

Chris came to the NIH at a time when the agency's mission was the subject of public debate. The NIH's funding came from the people, and therefore, some scientists argued, the money should be spent on basic research, studies that focused on fundamental scientific questions or tried to understand the processes that drove disease. Funding the research to turn ideas into drugs that could be used at a patient's bedside should be left up to the pharmaceutical companies, this line of argument went.

Chris knew from his own experiences that patients, especially those with rare diseases, could not rely on drug companies to find solutions for them. One only had to look at the statistics: there were around seven thousand known diseases that affected humans, and only five hundred had treatments. Many people were left without recourse or options.

"Companies can only work on projects that have a realistic chance of financial return in the relatively near term," Chris told me. "Most diseases are risky enough that a company can't see their way clear to work on the problem unless someone else does the de-risking."

The NIH could not turn itself into a drug developer, Chris recognized, but he wanted to create a place where scientists did enough work on promising drug leads to attract the attention of drug companies that could then take it from there, funding and running years-long clinical trials.

"The promise of genetics to deliver new interventions, new drugs, and new treatments for patients is not going to happen," Chris told his boss, "unless there is some way to get through the Valley of Death." Francis gave Chris a green light to pursue his vision.

CHRIS SET OUT TO BUILD a lab containing sophisticated equipment that could do rapid screening of drug libraries, enabling a more accelerated approach to identifying potential compounds to treat disease. In academic labs, scientists often had to do the work by hand, using pipettes to carefully measure chemicals into wells filled with a cell or protein that they wanted to try to fix. Big companies like Merck automated this type of work using robots that could search far more compounds at a much more rapid pace, but the cost was considered prohibitive for a single academic institution and many academic investigators still did things the old-fashioned way. Chris built a robotics system at the NIH lab that could do the type of automated screening typically employed at drug companies. It cost around $30 million, was fully automated, and included three robots that worked around-the-clock, twenty-four hours a day, seven days a week. Chris estimated the robots screened hundreds of thousands of compounds every day.

To do any drug search, researchers first created an assay, a test that included the proteins or cells involved in driving a disease. The robots could examine multiple different doses of the same drug at the same time. If one of the screened compounds registered a desired change or corrected a problem in the cells, the scientists could move the compound forward to a group of chemists who refined the drug even further. Unlike the scientists employed by drug companies, government researchers did not have to think about the commercial realities. They were mission-, not profit-, driven, and could keep experiments going, even in diseases with which the number of people affected was small.

To help spread the word about the lab, Chris spent a lot of time on the road traveling. He gave talks at universities, academic medical centers, and hospitals. He spoke about the challenges of drug development and how the robots might accelerate scientific projects, and encouraged scientists with a good idea to reach out. Chris figured that the people most likely to want to partner with NIH would be scientists working at universities or medical centers who didn't have access to the kinds of sophisticated screening technologies the new NIH lab boasted.

But increasingly, much to his surprise, Chris also fielded requests for help from people who were not scientists. Many of them barely recalled the fundamentals of their high school biology class but had turned themselves into experts on conditions most general practitioners never saw. At rare disease conferences, after Chris gave a talk, ordinary people with no scientific training at all frequently waited for the crowds to disperse so they could tell their stories to him. Some were parents of children with fatal diseases who had raised funds and were looking to support good ideas that might help their children and accelerate the development of a drug.

What became increasingly clear to Chris from interactions with these people was that patient advocates no longer depended solely on doctors for information. Through the internet, they could find one another and communicate. They swapped leads on clinicians who saw the most patients with a rare condition and offered suggestions to one another on how to better navigate social services. They downloaded scientific papers from the internet and reached out to the researchers to ask more questions.

Some of the advocates heard Chris and his team talk about the robots and figured it might be a way for them to get a drug developed. They started asking to visit the lab. Chris didn't turn them down. He often gave the tours himself, explaining how the robots and the automated system worked. He pointed out how the robots never got tired, their bright yellow arms keeping up a steady pace.

One day, Chris got a sobering reminder that technology alone was likely not enough to find cures in time for many of his visitors. The mother of a teenage boy with cancer was visiting doctors at the NIH and wanted to see the robots. Chris showed her how the robots moved the plastic plates of wells filled with different drugs from one station to the next. He gave her the standard pitch: We are going to disrupt the way science gets done; the robots can speed up the time it takes to develop a new drug. The mother asked by how much. Companies estimated the time from a lab to a patient was seventeen years, Chris said, but they thought they could do it in ten. The mother never took her eyes off the robots. "I love your technology, I love your robots, I love this fancy stuff," she told Chris. "But ten years isn't going to work. In ten years, my son could be dead."

CHRIS STARTED THINKING about the need to find novel ways to work with patients and advocates who, like that mother, operated with a sense of urgency and wanted to disrupt the system. He tried to approach building such a partnership like any other scientific problem, by devising a hypothesis and then setting out to test it.

The hypothesis was patients could help accelerate drug

development if they were involved in the process from the very beginning. It wasn't good enough to involve patients or advocates only when a company was ready to start enrolling them in a clinical trial. Patients should have a say in proposing what research questions got asked in the first place and, once there was data, an opportunity to contribute thoughts on which drug leads got prioritized to move forward.

Scientists didn't always want to work with patients or advocates in the early stages of a project, in part, Chris said, because "conventional wisdom is that patients impede the process."

One afternoon in his office, Chris put forth the case against collaboration that scientists often made. Patients did not have familiarity with science or scientific terms and concepts. They didn't know the regulatory rules. They did not fully appreciate the risks involved in trying experimental compounds. "Science demands a level of rigor and skepticism and a tolerance for failure that is difficult in the best of circumstances for scientists who really get devoted to what they do," Chris said. "The concern was if a patient was involved or a parent, it might not matter what the data showed. They would find it difficult to admit that the data were not promising because of wishful thinking."

Chris then turned around and argued the other side. Patients brought connections to the scientific community that were important. They knew the researchers in the field better than anyone. At critical moments, they were able to marshal support—raising funds for additional experiments, calling or meeting with their congressional representatives to draw public attention to inequities in research, appealing to the FDA to approve a drug—that could help keep an experiment going or launch the next one. They knew better than anyone how much was too much for a sick child to endure in order to participate in a clinical trial. Above all, Chris said, "They have a sense of urgency, a sense of focus and staying on task to get to a therapeutic outcome."

Chris wanted to build a scientific team consisting of patients and advocates and parents as well as scientists, clinicians, and researchers. Could professional scientists and citizen scientists work together as partners and combine their different types of expertise?

Scientists could never know the answer for sure unless they ran the experiment. Now all Chris needed was an opportunity to test the idea. He finally got the chance in November 2007.

More than a dozen people showed up for the meeting in Chris's lab to discuss the prospect of working together. Chris had already met many of the people in the room. One parent had been introduced to Chris months before by a scientist in the lab who gave a presentation at a lysosomal storage diseases conference. The parent approached the scientist to talk about developing drugs for NPC disease and ended up with an invitation to visit Chris's lab. Chris and Daniel Ory, the scientist who had traveled to Brazil, had been medical school classmates together. They had lost touch after their graduation. Chris and Marc Patterson were both neurologists who shared common scientific interests. Denny Porter was Chris's NIH colleague. Phil Marella, the parent of two children with NPC disease, had visited the NIH before as part of the natural history study. "The Hempels were the newbies," Chris said. The scientist ended up seated next to Chris Hempel during the meeting. He was amazed to learn that Addi and Cassi had been diagnosed just three weeks earlier. Chris was the father of three girls himself, and he marveled at the couple's resolve to attend a meeting about a novel scientific collaboration while still coming to terms with the shattering NPC diagnosis.

Chris sent out someone to pick up sandwiches, bags of potato chips, and cans of soda, and they got started. The goal, they soon agreed, was to find drugs that they could get into a clinical trial within three to five years. Chris agreed to use the robots to test thousands of different drugs on skin cells that Denny collected during the natural history study of children with NPC disease. Once they generated a list of promising drugs that got the cholesterol stuck in the cells moving again, they could winnow down the candidates and figure out which one to push forward.

During the discussion, Chris tried to highlight some of the potential scientific obstacles. The robots might generate any number of promising leads. The NPC collaborative did not have enough scientists, funding, or time to pursue them all. "You may need to choose," Chris reminded the group, and they could make the wrong choice, leaving them no better off than they had been before. "If you look at the history of medicine," Chris said, "you will find any number of examples where perfectly reasonable hypotheses turned out to be wrong in clinical trials."

Chris later worried that he should have talked more directly about the possibility of disagreements arising over their different views about the goals of science. He wondered if he should have forced everyone to draft some type of constitution laying out common principles. Even as an exercise, he thought, it could have identified areas where they might clash in the future. It wasn't simply that parents of seriously ill children with a fatal disease and scientists used to doing basic research in the lab might have different agendas. Chris's main worry was, "They have different belief systems." But Chris hesitated about interjecting such concerns at a time when everyone seemed united about the task ahead.

Later, Chris took the visitors to see the robots. Standing together, the parents and scientists watched as a robot claw added patients' cells to small plates, then moved them to another place in the work area where drugs and chemicals were added. During the tour, Chris Hempel asked Chris Austin whether they had named the robots yet. The scientist said they had not. "I have a name for you," Chris Hempel said. "I think you should name it Hope." After everyone left for the day, Chris stayed behind. He felt a similar surge of emotion that he sometimes got after performing in an opera. He didn't want to go home yet. Looking back on the day years later, he said, "I felt like we might actually be able to conquer this thing working together."

6

THE BROAD JUMP

Chris Hempel kept a running list of the leads the scientists were pursuing. She gleaned information from published studies. She dug into presentations of preliminary data shared at conferences. She also spent hours on the phone with the director of a patient advocacy group, poring over funded grant proposals, trying to figure out which ones seemed most promising.

She knew that scientists, not patients, traditionally came up with the ideas that got proposed to major funders like the NIH. Patient foundations might give out research grants, but they did not always have a master plan for moving a drug forward into clinical trials or the funding to support such a long and arduous effort. As a result, investigators typically pursued scientific theories and questions that caught their eye. The questions they asked might—or might not—have relevance for finding cures in the lifetimes of the patients struggling with a disease.

By the time she was done surveying the research landscape, Chris said, "I had fifteen different things on the list," but no clear path for saving her daughters.

Chris couldn't believe how much her life had changed in the weeks after getting back from the meeting at Chris Austin's lab at the NIH. Her days once consisted mainly of trips to the Baskin-Robbins ice cream shop, story hour with the girls at the library, and running errands at Walmart. Now Chris's mother moved into the house to help care for the girls. Chris's father lived in a small cottage set at the back of his daughter and son-in-law's property. Thirty years after their divorce, Chris's parents shared caregiving duties for their two granddaughters so Chris could spend more time tracking down leads.

She knew that the scientists worried about the parents moving too quickly to use a drug in the children before the researchers could figure out how or why it worked. If something went wrong in one child, the scientists warned, the event could potentially derail efforts to conduct experiments in the broader community down the road. Chris

Austin told the parents how he used to do the broad jump in high school. "You jump as far as you can in one step," he said. "You got eight feet instead of one." He reminded them, "Science is used to going in little baby steps. You know at every step what you're doing and it's very controlled." Despite the scientists' worries, Chris Hempel was determined to jump as far as she could go.

SHE SAW HER CHANCE almost immediately. A few weeks after she returned to Reno, one of the researchers sent Chris an early copy of a soon-to-be published paper that had many scientists in the community buzzing. Scientists at the University of Texas Southwestern Medical School in Dallas reported that the life span of mice treated with a single dose of a compound called cyclodextrin was extended by nearly 50 percent. The progressive loss of neurons that were a hallmark of the disease was also delayed, although not halted. The results were exciting, far better than any of the other promising drugs on Chris's list. Chris read the paper several times with growing excitement. This might very well be the drug they were all looking for, she thought.

Cyclodextrin had already been around for more than a century. The first mention appeared in an 1891 paper by a French scientist who observed a crystal-like substance growing on moldy bread but wasn't exactly sure what it was. Over the course of the next decades, scientists studied the substances, trying to understand their chemical structure. They eventually called them cyclodextrin, but it wasn't until the 1970s that manufacturers found a way to produce and market the compounds on an industrial scale. Once the chemical became more affordable, manufacturers started using cyclodextrin more routinely in a variety of products. Drug makers relied on cyclodextrin as an additive that helped stabilize drugs, enabling their injection into the bloodstream. Food manufacturers added them into butter and other dairy products to create low-cholesterol alternatives.

The new study—along with work published in 2009 by Albert Einstein College of Medicine scientist Steven Walkley's lab that demonstrated that the administration of cyclodextrin to the mice every other day provided even more benefit—raised the possibility of using cyclodextrin as a medicine, one that might successfully treat NPC disease.

The recognition of cyclodextrin's potential as a therapy came about serendipitously, when scientists were pursuing a different lead. Researchers originally noticed that the level of a neurosteroid vital for normal brain development—called allopregnanolone—dropped right before the onset of disease symptoms in NPC mice. The scientists then hypothesized they might be able to stop the progression of the disease by raising the level of allopregnanolone back to normal. The preliminary results were remarkable. Mice given a single dose of the steroid seven days after birth doubled their life span and exhibited a significant delay in the start and progression of neurological symptoms.

To ensure the results were valid and not simply due to chance, scientists in other labs ran comparison experiments. They gave some of the mice allopregnanolone. They also set up a so-called control arm. Animals in a control arm usually got something that was not expected to have any effect at all, such as saline solution. The results were then compared. These types of comparisons helped scientists better determine if an experimental therapy was truly making a difference in slowing down or stopping a disease's progression.

In the original study about allopregnanolone, the compound had been dissolved into cyclodextrin, in order to stabilize it. So for the control arm, the scientists trying to replicate the original study's results gave the mice cyclodextrin alone. They expected the animals receiving allopregnanolone with cyclodextrin to live longer than the mice getting only cyclodextrin.

Instead, the mice in the cyclodextrin group thrived. They got fatter, remained social, and continued to walk and move.

The scientists initially thought there was some kind of mistake. So they ran the experiment again with more mice. The benefits of cyclodextrin held.

The researchers did not understand how or why cyclodextrin was working. Over the years, different scientific groups conducted more experiments and demonstrated that cyclodextrin released the cholesterol from the part of the cell where it was trapped. But exactly how the compound successfully shuttled the cholesterol out is something scientists are trying to figure out even today.

Chris knew the results in the paper were preliminary and that the experiments had been conducted in mice. But the girls' condition weighed on her. Sometimes, Chris and Hugh watched old home movies of the girls singing the alphabet song in the bathtub, their faces covered with bubbles. They sobbed realizing the children couldn't do that anymore.

Chris wanted to talk to the scientists who wrote the paper. She called the lab and asked for Benny Liu, the author whose name was listed first. Benny, surprised to hear from a parent wanting details about one of his experiments, was curious and took the call.

Chris introduced herself and told the researcher about her twin girls, their fatal disease, and her efforts to find a drug to treat them. She explained that she wanted to apply the mice results to her children. "This is kind of crazy," Benny told Chris. "We still aren't really sure what is going on."

Every few weeks, Chris checked in. Benny updated her about the experiments. She sent photos of the girls. When they finally met for the first time in Tucson, Arizona, at the 2008 Parseghian Foundation scientific conference, they greeted each other like old friends. Benny said he would try to help Chris and the girls' doctor figure out a safe amount of cyclodextrin if she still wanted to test it in the girls. The scientists kept doing experiment after experiment, and the results gave Benny greater confidence that the drug was indeed extending the mice's life span and was safe to use. Benny met more parents and children at the conferences where he presented the mice data. He sympathized with their sense of urgency. "The girls don't have anything else," Benny said about why he agreed to help Chris. "They would die if we didn't try something."

Cyclodextrin wasn't available on pharmacy shelves, but there were companies around the world that manufactured and sold the compound for use by labs, companies, and re-searchers. Chris compiled a list of distributors and reached out to a small company in Florida whose owner agreed to help after hearing her story. "Cyclodextrin was something I could get my hands on," she said.

The FDA allowed physicians to request permission to try

experimental drugs in patients with lethal diseases through its expanded access, or compassionate use, program. Some of the scientists closest to Chris, including several participating in the recently formed collaborative with the parents, told her they thought it was too soon to seek such permission from the agency. The experiments showing that the drug extended the life span of the animals had been conducted in infant mice, seven days after they were born. Cyclodextrin did not demonstrate similar benefits in experiments involving older mice. When making comparisons, the children with NPC were at an age more comparable to the older mice. The scientists wanted to conduct additional experiments. In their view, the potential risks outweighed the benefits. They suggested to Chris that she wait—six more months, a year—for more data to become available. "We don't have a year to wait," Chris said. In that span of time, the girls' skills might degenerate even further. Chris and Hugh decided to ask Caroline Hastings, the twins' doctor, to move forward and seek FDA permission to give the girls cyclodextrin infusions.

CHRIS AND HUGH TRAVELED to New York City in early February 2009 for the latest meeting of the collaborative. When the couple arrived, they found Phil Marella, Cindy Parseghian, and several other parents crowded together on a sofa in the lobby. Chris pulled out a large sandwich she had bought on the way over. She unwrapped the aluminum foil and held it out to the other parents. "Does anyone want to share?" she asked. The other parents smiled but didn't take her up on the offer.

The scientists were already in a conference room talking privately. Daniel Ory, Steven Walkley, Denny Porter, and other scientists involved in NPC research wanted to discuss the data from their latest experiments before meeting with the parents. Around twenty minutes later, a woman led the parents to their own conference room. As the parents headed to the elevator, they walked past the glass-walled room where the scientists were already working. A whiteboard stood near one corner. Empty soda bottles and coffee cups were scattered across the table. The researchers were so intent on discussing the data from their various experiments, they didn't look up as the parents walked by.

In their own meeting, the parents shared photos and updates about their children. But in a sign of how they had changed, the conversation quickly turned to science. They talked about a recent presentation of cyclodextrin data at a lysosomal storage disease conference. The results indicated that different formulations of the compound might affect the results. The parents had asked the scientists to run their own experiments to try to sort it out.

Cindy Parseghian informed the others that the foundation had received more applications than the year before from scientists interested in pursuing NPC research. She attributed the rise to the heightened awareness in the broader scientific community about NPC disease thanks to the NIH robot screening and the publication of the cyclodextrin studies.

So when the parents finally joined the scientists to discuss next steps, they were surprised to hear that Denny Porter, the NIH doctor, was hoping to start a clinical trial in children with NPC disease by the end of the year, but that the drug would not be cyclodextrin.

Scientists were used to being the ones in charge of picking the best drug to test in a clinical trial. Chris and Hugh had always hoped that by moving forward with testing cyclodextrin in their children, they might persuade the scientists to follow their lead, not the other way around. But when it came to cyclodextrin, Denny wasn't fully convinced.

Denny also did not yet want to share the name of the drug he preferred. But he told the group that the drug had promising results in mice. The results were not as good as those using cyclodextrin, he acknowledged to them, but the drug's safety profile was far better understood.

His reservations about cyclodextrin weren't only that

the drug might not work and the children would not benefit, Denny explained to them. They also needed to consider the possibility that using the drug could make things worse. What if the drug sped up the disease process and the children died even sooner than they otherwise would have? What if the parents moved too soon on cyclodextrin when something better was out there?

Denny worried that if the Hempels moved forward with cyclodextrin, then other parents, also impatient about the slower pace of science, might follow their lead and file compassionate use requests with the FDA to give the drug to their children. In his opinion, if the group wanted to pursue a path likeliest to eventually lead to an FDA drug approval, they needed to test the drug through a traditional clinical trial, not a group of compassionate use experiments.

In a community where the number of children potentially eligible to join any clinical trial might not top fifty, he cautioned the parents that even a handful of children getting the drug through compassionate use now would likely make it harder to draw enough patients for enrollment in a clinical trial later. A clinical trial was the best way to conclusively determine if the drug worked, he emphasized, and if it did, to seek FDA approval.

"I owe it to the kids to take it through the clinical trial process and say it truly does work or it doesn't work,"

Denny said. It was too soon to start a community-wide cyclodextrin trial.

CHRIS AND HUGH STILL WANTED to move forward. Caroline, Addi and Cassi's doctor, had agreed to help them, but she reminded the Hempels that the case for cyclodextrin largely rested on mice data. A mouse's brain was probably the size of a thumbnail, while a child's brain was larger than a softball. Taking a drug straight from a mouse to a child was a big leap. Usually, the FDA wanted some evidence the drug worked in larger animals such as dogs or cats or had been tried before in people.

Chris dug further into the history of cyclodextrin, searching for any information that might bolster their case. She came across a short report published in a medical journal years before. The patient was a child with a genetic condition that made it difficult to properly process vitamin A. The child's doctor gave the child an infusion of cyclodextrin in order to successfully remove the toxic buildup. Chris tracked down the doctor, who was still practicing medicine. He shared with her the safety data he gathered but reminded her it was from only a single patient.

Chris learned from one of the cyclodextrin suppliers that Janssen Pharmaceuticals, a subsidiary of Johnson & Johnson, used cyclodextrin as an additive in an FDA-approved drug to treat fungal infections in children and adults. As part of the FDA approval process for the antifungal drug, the company ran safety studies on the additive, cyclodextrin. The data could be invaluable in demonstrating that cyclodextrin could be safely taken by people. But all the information that companies file with the FDA during the drug approval process was considered confidential. The FDA was not allowed to dip into files belonging to one group in order to support another without the company's permission. Chris called Janssen's headquarters in Europe. The woman who took the call seemed perplexed by why the mother of sick children was seeking access to company drug files and told Chris she couldn't assist her. Chris decided to take another approach. This time, she wrote a letter to Janssen's parent company, Johnson & Johnson. "Dear Johnson & Johnson," she wrote, "do kids really matter to you?"

She explained that the information in the drug files could help save the lives of Addi and Cassi and other children afflicted with Niemann-Pick disease type C. She asked the company to give the FDA permission to use the data when considering Addi and Cassi's compassionate use request. When she was done, she posted the letter online on her blog.

Steven Silber, then a senior executive at the Johnson & Johnson division in charge of the antifungal drug, was out to dinner with his wife that Friday night for an early Valentine's Day celebration when his boss emailed him about

Chris's post. The next morning, the executive called the Hempels and woke the couple up. "I want to know about the girls," he told them. "I want to help."

Over the weekend, the company's regulatory affairs team identified the documents containing the cyclodextrin human safety data. They sent a letter to the FDA giving the agency permission to use the relevant sections when weighing the Hempels' petition. The next month, the FDA approved the family's compassionate use request.

AS THE DAY of the first infusion drew closer, Chris and Hugh's emotions vacillated between hope and fear. "You always worry that something bad could happen," Chris said.

Pharmacists created a sterile liquid solution safe enough to infuse into the girls. Doctors arranged for special equipment in the girls' room, in case the twins went into shock after receiving the infusion and the medical team had to try to save their lives.

The Hempels wanted to collect as much information as possible before the girls received the first infusion. Doctors took blood, urine, and stool samples. They measured the size of the girls' spleens and livers. They gave them a battery of cognitive tests. Researchers could study the data, Chris said. They might learn new things about the disease. Or perhaps, Chris told some of the other parents during their weekly calls, the information might someday prove useful to the FDA after all.

Chris had trouble sleeping the night before the infusion. In the morning, she and Hugh lifted the girls out of bed and put them in the car, still dressed in their matching pink nightgowns. "I don't know what is going to happen," Chris said.

At the hospital, the nurses pushed the twins' beds together. Chris crawled into the middle. She tucked each girl into the crook of an arm, lowered her head. She kissed each of them in turn, her face pressed on the top of the girls' heads, breathing in their scent. Addi and Cassi were quiet. They cuddled with their mother. Each girl would receive the cyclodextrin solution, now hanging in clear bags on poles next to their beds, through intravenous infusion. The children didn't seem to notice the quicksilver ministrations of the nurses, who got everything ready, or the rising emotions of the adults crowded in the room. When the infusions finally got underway, the girls still didn't make a sound. It was Chris who started to cry.

7

NEW HIT

The parents and scientists returned to Chris Austin's lab in November 2009 for the latest gathering of the collaborative. It felt momentous to be back in the same place where they had first met, trying to imagine a new way to work together.

The meeting had been called to discuss the potential candidates that might eventually be part of a drug cocktail to treat NPC disease. They still hoped to get their first candidate into trial by 2011. But as the day got underway, it quickly became apparent that the parents and scientists disagreed on what direction to go.

From Chris Hempel's perspective, the first iteration of

the drug cocktail already existed. Her daughters were receiving twice-a-week cyclodextrin intravenous infusions as well as daily Zavesca pills, the drug that many NPC doctors prescribed off-label. Now Chris and some of the other parents planned to ask the scientists to seek a federal research grant to support experiments in the lab and animals that might allow them to make the case to the FDA for the launch of a cyclodextrin trial.

As everyone settled in and found their seats, Chris Hempel gave Chris Austin a smile. "Hugh cut my hair," Chris told the scientist. The long black hair Chris wore all her life was gone. In its place, she now sported a pixie cut.

"I didn't recognize you at first," Chris Austin said with a laugh.

Chris had been coloring her hair for years, but since the girls' diagnosis, she rarely got to the hair salon. One August evening, Chris and Hugh headed to a friend's house for a fiftieth birthday party. Chris wore a hat to hide the big white streak down the middle of her hair. The couple drank wine and enjoyed the party. But later that evening, Chris stood in front of the bathroom mirror holding scissors in one hand and her hair in the other. Her old life was gone. She made the first cut. By the time Hugh stirred and came into the bathroom to see what was happening, Chris's shorn hair was piling up on the counter. "Let me help you," Hugh offered quietly. He put a towel down on the bathroom floor and used hair clippers to cut the rest. All that remained when he was finished was a quarter inch of gray fuzz, Chris recounted.

Chris was starting to get used to her new self. The hair had grown in, and a hair stylist had shaped it into the pixie cut. Chris wore jeans and a maroon hoodie to the meeting but had also decided to put on a pair of heels. Even so, she knew she could never go back to the way things had been before, she told the scientist.

THE PARENTS WORKED CLOSELY with the scientists to create an initial list of around fifty compounds to test on Chris Austin's robots. They had all made suggestions, identifying leads from multiple sources. The parents drew some ideas from the scientific literature not only about NPC disease but also other neurological conditions that shared some common symptoms, such as Alzheimer's disease. The scientists mined their own work and that of their colleagues.

Chris Hempel started looking more closely at the results on a chart the Austin lab created for the presentation. Her eyes went immediately to the names that might address the accumulation of cholesterol in the NPC cells. Rapamycin, curcumin, lovastatin—all familiar names from the group's previous conversations. Then Chris noticed something unusual. One promising lead had no name. On the chart the mystery compound had been labeled, "NIH New Hit."

One of the scientists in Chris Austin's lab stood in the front of the room getting ready to present an overview of the findings when Chris Hempel called out to him, "What's the drug's name?"

The scientist looked uncomfortable but didn't answer the question. Instead, he told Chris, "We'll talk later."

WHEN THE FIRST DAY'S presentations were over, everyone gathered together in a conference room for a toast. The parents arranged to bring in wine and a platter of food. People filled plastic cups with wine and served themselves cheese, artichokes, salami, and peppers. Despite the tension of the day, they had sat as partners at the same table. A hush fell over the room as one of the parents raised a glass to mark the moment. "To the scientists who are doing God's work for our children," the parent said. "We're so grateful." Everyone took a drink. "And to our children," the parent added. Everyone raised their glasses again.

"And to the parents who inspire us," said Steven Walkley, one of the scientists who had helped found the collaborative, offering a toast on behalf of the scientists.

"Well, I wasn't going to say it," the parent replied, "but I'm glad you did." Everyone laughed.

Afterward, Chris slipped away. She wanted to talk to the scientist who gave the NIH's presentation. She was determined not to end the first day of the meeting without knowing the name of New Hit.

THE PARENTS HAD AGREED to gather in the bar of the hotel where they were all staying to assess the day's events when Chris came racing in. Only one other parent had arrived. But Chris felt like she couldn't wait another moment to share what she'd learned. "I think I am going to cry," she said, and threw her arms around the parent's neck. He hugged her and asked her what was wrong. Chris's voice trembled when she said, "Do you know what it is? Do you know the name?"

Chris didn't need to explain. They both knew she was talking about New Hit. "It's vitamin E, vitamin E, vitamin E!" she exclaimed. "When were they planning on telling us? When our kids are dead?"

Over the din of the bar, Chris gave a short summary of what had happened. The scientist told Chris he sympathized with her desire to know the name, but the NIH team had decided they didn't feel comfortable sharing the information until they had completed more experiments. Yes, in their first experiments, the compound appeared to correct the problem in the cells. But that was a long way from knowing that they could find a way to deliver the drug into the brains of the children, or that the drug was safe, and would have the same effect in living children as it did in cells in a lab. Those were the scientific reasons, but there were also other considerations. The team did not want to publicly announce the drug's name until they could apply for a patent. A patent was crucial in order for the NIH to stake a claim to the discovery, the scientist explained.

The goal of the collaboration was to find promising drugs and rapidly advance their development to the point that drug companies might want to step in. But drug companies had boards and investors to whom they had to answer. They wouldn't take the risk of investing tens of millions of dollars in commercializing a drug if the NIH didn't have a patent securing the rights to the intellectual property.

Chris took in all the scientist said. She told him that she understood his reasons. But, she added, she still wanted to know. From her perspective, sharing the name of New Hit was a test of the collaboration. Did the scientists truly believe in the revolutionary concept that parents and scientists could work as equal partners, each offering their essential expertise and their particular set of values? If they did, then the partnership included weighing the evidence and making judgments together about what drugs should go forward. How could they devise such a strategy if only some of the people involved had access to all the information? In the end, the scientist told Chris the name. New Hit was a form of vitamin E known as delta-tocopherol.

"I wasn't sure I wanted to know the name until the scientists are ready," the parent told Chris.

"We started this collaboration to find and use off-the-shelf drugs," Chris said. "Now we are talking about patents and papers."

"We can't just criticize the system," the parent replied. "We have to offer an alternative."

THE NEXT DAY, Chris offered a vision of one possible alternative. The scientists should keep studying New Hit. The data were promising but might require months of additional experiments before the scientists knew for sure if the compound should be a leading candidate for the cocktail. Meanwhile, a short-term project should also move ahead. Chris's daughters were receiving cyclodextrin through the compassionate use program. Other parents were also considering seeking permission from the FDA to use the drug. The collaborative should set up a way to collect data from the compassionate use cases and seek an FDA-sponsored grant to gather more. By definition, such a project would likely involve only a small number of children. Not all parents would want to be involved given the unknown risks and benefits. But even if the compassionate use studies contained only a handful of children, if the data was gathered in a standardized way, it might be more useful to their long-term goal of creating a drug cocktail than continuing with testing compounds only in the lab or in mice.

"I'm going to cut to the chase," another parent added after Chris threw out her idea. "We don't want a one-off effort on cyclodextrin. We want to integrate it into everything else. How should we proceed?"

But the scientists, even those most excited about the potential of cyclodextrin, said they still didn't know enough about the drug to seek funding for such a study. They had no reliable way to measure if the drug was working. In an ongoing cyclodextrin study involving cats, two of the animals had suddenly died. And despite the improvements and changes Chris noticed in her children, "That's not enough to say scientifically speaking that any change is not due to chance," Daniel Ory said.

AT THE END of the meeting, Chris Austin asked two of the scientists in the collaborative—Daniel Ory and Steven Walkley—to test New Hit in their labs. By dividing up the experiments, Chris hoped the scientists could figure out more quickly the best drug to take into a trial. But the tension over New Hit lingered. Chris Austin worried that in the future, the collaboration might not look the same.

After the meeting, Chris Hempel boarded her flight back to Reno thinking something similar. A few weeks after Hugh cut her hair, he came to pick her up after an outing. Chris saw him waiting and waved, trying to get her husband's attention. Hugh stared right at her but gave no sign he recognized her. Later, she asked him what had happened. "He was looking for a different Chris," she said.

8

REVERBERATIONS

Phil Marella prepared carefully for his appearance at the FDA advisory committee meeting held on a brisk January day in 2010. He honed his speech, incorporating feedback from a friend who worked in public relations on how to sharpen his message. He practiced out loud to make sure he kept his remarks to within the seven-minute time limit, even though he had a lot more to say. He packed a nice suit, pairing it with a crisp blue shirt and a bold red tie. Phil intended to be seen. Even more, he wanted to be heard.

The hearing, held in a quotidian conference room of a Silver Spring, Maryland, hotel, had been convened at the

FDA's request. The biotech company Actelion wanted the regulators to approve the company's drug Zavesca to treat people with Niemann-Pick disease type C. If the agency eventually signed off, Zavesca would become the first FDA-approved treatment for the condition.

But the drug's approval was not a certainty. For one thing, FDA regulators sent a memo to members of the advisory panel stating that a reason for holding the hearing was that the clinical trial failed to meet its initial objective of improving patients' rapid eye movements. The data, they said, did not reveal a significant difference in outcome between patients taking the drug and those who did not. But the agency did not immediately reject the company's request for approval. NPC was a lethal disease without any effective treatments. The trial generated data about changes in other symptoms too, such as the patients' swallowing and speech. And in those areas, some people on the drug showed signs of improvement. Were the results enough to merit the approval of the drug? The agency wasn't sure. It wanted advice from the panel, comprised of doctors and scientists and one patient advocate. Patients and families also got invited to speak.

For years, ever since the neurologist Marc Patterson wrote off-label prescriptions for Zavesca to treat the Marella children, Phil noticed its effect on their symptoms. Dana Marella started taking Zavesca when she was eleven years old, after she had already lost the ability to walk or talk. Her younger brother, Andrew, who was tested after his sister's diagnosis, had been taking the drug since the age of five, before overt signs of the disease emerged. Six years later, Andrew still lived a normal life. He struggled in math and some other subjects, but he attended regular school with friends in the neighborhood. He could still walk and run. Phil attributed the differences between the two siblings to the fact that Andrew started taking Zavesca earlier in the progression of the disease. "You look at Dana and you look at Andrew and I realize every kid can be different, but give me a break," Phil said. "There is no comparison. I believe Zavesca is beneficial for my kids. The question is how do we prove it?"

That question weighed not only on the parents and scientists regarding Zavesca, but also for every drug that might come after it—most especially cyclodextrin.

Phil and other parents held regular catch-up calls, always checking in about one another's children before turning to the project of how to move science and drug development forward more quickly. Chris Hempel told the group that her girls appeared to benefit from their regular cyclodextrin infusions. They fell down less, Chris said, and had fewer bruised knees. The children seemed more engaged and energetic when interacting with each other and with other family members. Phil found the observations compelling. No one was more attuned to changes in children's behavior and health than their parents, or better practiced in assessing what counted as an improvement in the quality of their lives.

But he also knew that if the NIH or a biotech company or even a group of parents wanted to someday get FDA approval for cyclodextrin, regulators required more than personal observations.

In some diseases, it was easier to assess if a drug was helping patients. Someone with lung disease could breathe in a special tube to measure lung function. A patient taking a drug to improve blindness could be asked to try to read an eye chart. Patients with NPC disease suffered a variety of different symptoms, which might emerge at different times through their lives. A child might walk well but be unable to speak clearly. Another could appear shaky on his feet but recite jokes by heart from a popular sitcom. Drugs like Zavesca—or cyclodextrin—didn't fix the underlying gene defect that caused the disease. Some patients were diagnosed as infants; others did not receive a diagnosis until later in childhood or early adulthood, when it was more unlikely that an intervention might reverse the disease's damage. In trying to design a clinical trial, it was a challenge to pull from such wide-ranging experiences one major symptom to track and measure in order to demonstrate a drug's efficacy in a trial. A scientist involved in designing the Zavesca trial said, "We basically had to guess." In the end, even with promising drugs, scientists worried they might miss the benefits of a treatment not because the drug did not work, but because they chose the wrong outcome to measure.

ONCE THE ADVISORY hearing was underway, Phil could tell right away things were not going the way he wanted. An FDA scientist spoke first and questioned everything from the design of the trial to the significance of the results. Some patients reported walking better after a year on the drug. Others said their swallowing was better. But none of the results happened in enough patients to reach the statistical goals the company set out to prove. On all the measures they chose to prove the drug's efficacy, the company fell short.

The parents milled around the room during a break in the presentations. They seemed dejected by the criticism of the Zavesca results. "I told you we should have brought the tomatoes," Phil joked to one of the other parents. From their perspective, the entire morning had been about Zavesca's weaknesses and the trial design's flaws. In the afternoon, when the parents were scheduled to speak, the panel would finally hear testimony about the drug's benefits, insights based on the patients' lived experiences.

"I didn't expect it to feel like that much of an uphill battle," Phil said. He decided to retreat to his hotel room, skipping lunch so he could practice his speech again. "I need to practice, practice, practice," Phil said. "This is the most important speech of my life."

Phil called his wife, Andrea, who had missed the morning's scientific presentations in order to go sightseeing with their four children. He told her that when he addressed the committee, he didn't just want them in the audience, he wanted them standing next to him at the dais. "We didn't plan at first for all of us to go up there," Phil said, "but we needed to make an impact."

Andrea assured him they would all be there. Later she observed, "I have never seen him so nervous in his life."

WHEN IT WAS THE PARENTS' turn to address the panel, there was a change in the room. Panel members leaned forward, intent on hearing the parents' words. There was an energy that seemed absent when the scientists argued with one another over the data. Dillon Papier, a child with NPC disease who was taking Zavesca, sat quietly curled in his mother's lap for much of the morning's testimony. Now, as one parent after another came forward to talk, he jumped up and started walking up and down the aisle, slowly, shakily, but on his own. It was hard to know if Dillon was bored or if he wanted to tell the panel members something. As he walked back and forth, the boy raised the baseball he held in his hand to the light, like a beacon.

When it was Phil's turn, Andrea and the four children gathered around him. Don't base Zavesca's fate only on the results of the patients' eye movements, Phil urged. Consider the totality of his children's lives when measuring the effectiveness of the drug. "I don't think that when you are talking about people's health that you take eye movement as the measurement and end point and when that doesn't work you throw away the other evidence," Phil said.

Wasn't it important that Andrew got a high score on the school quiz listing the capitals of every state? Didn't the committee members notice that Dana, seated in a wheelchair, reached out to rub her younger brother Andrew's arm while their father talked? Dana's disease was advanced, but she remained actively engaged with her family. Phil considered such milestones the benefits of Zavesca.

"Zavesa hasn't stopped the progression of the disease in Dana. It hasn't stopped the progression in Andrew. But we are giving these kids more time. As a parent, you don't care if it is an hour, a day, or a week. The longer, the better," Phil said.

Before Phil or Andrea went to bed at night, they rotated Dana in her bed. Then they got up two hours later to turn Dana again. They did this a few times a night. They changed her position to prevent bedsores and because they felt it improved her breathing. "When we're in there taking care of Dana, she knows her mom and dad are taking care of her. She wakes up a bit, opens her eyes. She gives you a big smile. She reaches out a hand to hold your hand," Phil said. "Every extra day I get of that is a blessing."

At the end of a long day of testimony, the advisory panel debated whether to recommend that the FDA regulators approve Zavesca.

They struggled with the data, which they said often seemed like a set of subjective observations rather than concrete measurements. Perhaps the stability in the swallowing of some patients was not because they took Zavesca, but because the disease progressed more slowly in those particular patients.

The parents' observations about the difference Zavesca made in their children's lives constituted evidence of the benefits of taking the drug, a panel member countered.

"You hear very touching comments about how patients improve," one member of the panel said. "That's hard to ignore, but it's not science. When you look at the science, it falls short."

"I feel Zavesca is doing something," another offered, "but feelings are feelings, and if we vote on feelings, we vote on emotions, not science."

At one point, the panel members tried to parse what the

regulations meant when they stated "substantial evidence" was necessary in order to conclude that a drug worked. How much latitude did they all have in interpreting if the data before them that day even met that bar? "I'm not convinced it makes sense to use the same standard in rare diseases," one of the doctors on the panel pointed out.

They understood that their decision about Zavesca might have consequences that reverberated beyond the hotel conference room. If the panel voted that day to recommend that the FDA approve a drug based on negative clinical trial data but positive testimony from parents, it could set a precedent. Another company, with a different drug for some other disease and perhaps flimsier evidence, might someday stand in front of an FDA advisory panel and argue that if Zavesca merited FDA approval so did their drug. It was hard to know where to draw the line, they said.

The time to vote finally arrived. On the question of whether the trial showed that the drug worked, the majority of panel members voted no. The most crucial question came next: Should they recommend that the FDA approve Zavesca? Phil put his arms around another father with an NPC child who was sitting next to him. He bent his head and kept his eyes tightly shut, waiting. Phil opened his eyes only after the final tally was announced and he knew that in a vote of ten to three, the panel members recommended that the FDA approve the drug.

Phil tried to savor the moment, but he understood the victory could be temporary. The FDA might not accept the panel's recommendation. (In fact, a couple of months later, the FDA announced it was rejecting Actelion's request to approve the drug for NPC.)

The bar for FDA drug approval seemed hard to meet, especially for a disease as rare and complex as NPC. The Zavesca clinical trial had been sponsored by a drug company, designed by a top NPC neurologist, and supported by the patient community. Despite a significant investment of resources, the company still hadn't managed to gather enough persuasive data to convince the FDA. "If they don't approve this, then what about cyclodextrin?" Phil said, a drug far less studied than Zavesca. Phil didn't want cyclodextrin to end up in the same situation as Zavesca, with the FDA uncertain if the drug worked. The scientists needed time to choose the best trial design to ensure a clear result. Parents had to find a way to standardize the collection of data about the children who got the drug through compassionate use so the FDA would count it as scientific evidence. "You can't just sit there and say, 'My kids are better,'" Phil said.

ONCE THE HEARING CONCLUDED, the hotel room cleared out. The cleaning crew arrived, quickly putting away chairs, collecting abandoned coffee cups, restoring order. The parents did not want to immediately part ways. In a corner of the room, they gathered together. Denny Porter came over to join them. He had attended the hearing hoping to gain insights into the way FDA regulators and advisers measured benefit in drugs to treat NPC disease, and to support the parents and their children, his patients. He knew how important it was to the community to get Zavesca approved. Without FDA approval, some insurers refused to cover the cost of using Zavesca off-label in NPC children, even when doctors believed the children benefited and prescribed the drug. An FDA drug approval also represented a sign of hope to the community that things were going to change. Once the FDA approved one drug for treating NPC disease, they figured it was more likely other companies would follow and try to develop more.

Phil asked Denny for his assessment of the day's outcome. The parents' testimony made a difference, the doctor said. "The three who voted no voted on the science," Denny said. "The ten who voted yes voted on the parents."

Dillon stood at the edge of the circle. He wanted to talk to Denny too. At first, Dillon waited patiently for a turn. Then, he couldn't wait any longer. "Dr. Porter, Dr. Porter," Dillon called, trying to get the doctor's attention. Denny crouched down to greet Dillon, opening his arms wide for a hug. Dillon propelled himself into the doctor's arms. The force of Dillon's embrace caught Denny by surprise, knocking them both down. Tumbling, they bumped a table, where a tray of water glasses rested. The glasses jostled and shook. For a moment, it seemed like the tray might fall. Denny sat on the floor, the boy still in his arms. The other parents formed a circle around them. They waited together for the reverberations to stop.

9

PERSUASION

Chris and Hugh knew that their children were involved in an experiment. They tried to gather as much information as they could. Every morning, they woke at 4:00 a.m. in order to collect Addi's and Cassi's first-of-the-morning urine samples, which were sent to a lab for testing levels of proteins that might indicate irregularities in kidney function. The twins underwent regular imaging exams of their spleens and livers. Doctors examined them for any changes in gait, cognition, hearing, and muscle tone. All of the data were reported to the FDA as part of the conditions for using the drug.

"I'm waiting for the first scientist to acknowledge the

fact that the data that comes out of Addi and Cassi's experiences will be hugely valuable to the community," Hugh said one day after the couple returned from the latest cyclodextrin infusion at the hospital. "No one has come forward to say the data are important."

Then, in early 2010, Chris saw an opportunity to make her case. An announcement on the FDA website caught her eye. The agency's Office of Orphan Products Development was hosting a two-day workshop in February in Claremont, California—part of a broader effort to encourage companies and investigators to file more orphan drug designation applications.

An orphan drug designation was a key step in securing benefits for developing drugs for rare diseases. The Orphan Drug Act, passed by Congress in 1983 due to the efforts of patient advocates, provided drug companies with incentives to develop therapies for rare diseases. Companies received tax credits and a seven-year period to exclusively market an approved drug. But in order to qualify for the benefits, the FDA had to first grant the compound an orphan drug designation.

The prospect of the workshop gave Chris an idea. She could file an orphan drug designation for cyclodextrin under the sponsorship of the twins' doctor and the doctor's hospital. As part of the application process, the FDA would review the cyclodextrin data that the scientists had generated so far in the mice and cats. Chris also intended to include the girls' cyclodextrin data in the application. The FDA's imprimatur might help Chris finally convince the scientists in the collaboration that her girls' real-world cyclodextrin trial was also generating useful scientific knowledge alongside the more traditional animal studies. Parents like Chris didn't ordinarily get an opportunity to meet face-to-face with the FDA to discuss developing a drug. Companies or academic investigators were the ones typically expected to seek regulators' advice. Chris saw a chance to bypass the usual way things were done in science and go directly to the FDA regulators herself. She registered for the workshop and booked a flight to Southern California.

THE FDA WORKSHOP convened at the Keck Graduate Institute in Claremont. Small tables and benches were scattered outside in an open courtyard where people gathered for meals, taking in a view of the mountains. The company representatives participating in the workshop were a tight-lipped group. They did not want potential competitors to know anything about their products. Recognizing the need for privacy, the FDA went to great lengths to protect people's identities. Name badges contained first names only. When people introduced themselves, they did not share last names, titles, or company affiliations. Each group was assigned a number, and the numeral was the only identification that appeared outside the rooms where they met with their designated FDA advisers.

At meals, people rarely mingled. For the most part, those present congregated with their colleagues. If someone new joined a table they asked permission before sitting down and kept any conversation innocuous, general, and polite. People largely stuck to discussing the weather or the prospects of a sports team.

Chris ignored the instructions. She was animated and outgoing and hard to miss at the conference. She dressed in jeans, heels, and a long sweater. After boarding the buses that shuttled people from the hotel to the workshop and back again, Chris plunked herself down on any open seat and cheerfully introduced herself to her neighbors. She wrote her first and last name on her conference badge. Chris and Hugh had recently joined a group of parents and friends of children with rare diseases in jump-starting a new advocacy group called Global Genes. Unlike many organizations, Global Genes focused not on advancing research in one disease, but rather on helping parents and families more effectively navigate the drug development space and accelerate therapies for their children and others with rare diseases. At the FDA workshop, Chris decided to promote the group's mission. She handed out to befuddled participants small ribbons the color of denim blue jeans, attached to a small card that read, "Hope, it's in our genes." The others did not quite know what to make of her or the gesture, turning over the cards with quizzical expressions. "Who are you?" one young man asked Chris. He wasn't wearing a name badge, defiant in maintaining his anonymity. "I'm a mom," Chris said. He tucked the card inside his jacket and scurried away.

At the first day's introductory session, the twenty-nine participants gathered together. The FDA, they were told, decided to send regulators into the field to drum up orphan drug designation applications. They hoped to double the number of applications for orphan drug designations. More applications might eventually result in more approved drugs to treat rare diseases. "We're barely scratching the surface," the FDA official told them.

Participants needed to provide evidence that a drug showed some promise of working. And the FDA was increasingly open to multiple ways to demonstrate promise. These days, the agency accepted all kinds of data. A clinical trial, if one had already been run. Case reports from doctors about an unusual patient. Animal studies with interesting results. The important thing, the official urged, was to submit "data, not whimsical theories."

Chris's hand immediately shot up. She wanted to know what advantages an orphan drug designation offered to a patient advocate, especially when the drug in question was not yet pursued for commercial development by any company. An orphan drug designation was a key to unlock money, attention, pharmaceutical company interest, the FDA official replied—in other words, credibility. "It signifies the FDA has given a nod that this compound has promise and may be effective. That tends to get things rolling." Chris gave a smile. That was exactly why she was there.

After the opening remarks, the teams went in separate directions. Each group was assigned to an FDA adviser, who offered feedback and suggestions about how to fill out a successful application. Chris entered a small, claustrophobic room and folded herself into a chair. The FDA official sat behind a small desk. She introduced herself as Marilyn and said she had worked in various capacities at the FDA for the past ten years. Her short hair was the color of burnt oranges, and she wore a cross encrusted with small stones that glittered. She held out her hands for the stack of paper Chris had gathered, a short history about the promise of cyclodextrin.

For the first time since Chris began her foray into the world of drug development, she seemed nervous, even a bit tentative. She blurted out to Marilyn that she was not a scientist, but a mother of twins. She wondered how receptive the FDA would be to the claims of a mother rather than a drug company. "We are in a tricky situation," Chris told Marilyn.

"The process is still the same," Marilyn reassured her. If Chris could prove that cyclodextrin showed promise, if she could persuade the FDA of the drug's merit, the orphan drug designation was hers. Marilyn reminded Chris that it was not enough to state that cyclodextrin might work; Chris needed a way to document the scientific rationale behind her claim.

"We have scientific papers," Chris said. "We have animal data. We have my girls."

With the mention of her children, the reason for Chris's presence in that room suddenly came into sharper focus. It wasn't enough that a year earlier the FDA had approved the Hempel family's compassionate use request enabling cyclodextrin infusions for the girls. To many in the community, the FDA decision was an act of sympathy toward the desperate parents of two fatally ill children, justified by morality more than by science. The designation, on the other hand, involved a dispassionate weighing of the evidence. As Marilyn pointed out, they needed data demonstrating a scientific basis for thinking cyclodextrin might work. To Chris, the designation was not only a statement about cyclodextrin's value, but an assessment of her own scientific acumen, that what she had done with the girls was not a last-ditch effort by parents willing to try anything, but a reasonable action based on the weighing of the scientific facts at hand.

Marilyn carefully scrutinized each page. When she was done, she looked up at Chris. Everything looked good, she declared, but she still needed a key item before filing the application: a binder to hold all the documents.

When the meeting ended, Chris drove to the nearest Staples. In the middle of the day, the store wasn't busy. Chris stood next to a wall of binders in an array of colors, considering her options: red, brown, black, navy blue, the binders lined up like soldiers. Black or navy would have been the more traditional choice. But pink was the girls' favorite color. "It is a lucky color," she said.

Chris liked to imagine a curious regulator plucking her binder out to read first, a pink buoy in a churning sea of dull navy blue and black binders. "I wonder if the FDA has ever received a filing in a pink binder," Chris said, and filled up the cart.

SHE ARRIVED BACK in time for the afternoon review session with Marilyn. Marilyn didn't say a word about the binder's unusual color or look surprised when Chris pulled a small video camera out of her bag to record the scene. Chris turned the lens on Marilyn as the other woman went over the documents again, one final check. Everything, it seemed, was finally in order. The orphan drug designation request, Marilyn declared, was officially ready for submission. "We're kind of giddy over here," Chris said.

Marilyn looked directly into the camera and offered a small smile. "Your hard work is paying off," she told Chris.

The FDA approved the orphan drug designation for cyclodextrin three months later. Marilyn had told Chris that companies often marked the occasion with a press release. Chris decided to share the milestone on her blog. "Drum roll, please!" she wrote, and spread the news.

CHRIS SOON LEARNED that in the debate over what drug to push forward into a clinical trial, cyclodextrin started to take the lead. She couldn't help but hope that the granting of the orphan drug designation had helped make a difference.

At the NIH, Chris Austin reviewed all the scientific evidence to date. Denny Porter had enrolled thirty NPC patients in the clinical trial he promised the parents at the meeting in New York, testing N-acetyl cysteine, a widely available antioxidant. Denny told parents who asked why he needed to test something they could already buy in a store: even the most innocuous-seeming drug could have unexpected outcomes. His warning was borne out when some patients in the trial experienced spikes in their liver enzymes, a potential warning sign the drug might damage the organ. The delta-tocopherol experiments Chris Austin requested also hadn't panned out. The NPC mice weren't getting better. Chris knew that because the NIH would be the main funder of any clinical trial, his word carried weight on what to do next. But after more than three years of working closely with the parents, he didn't want to make the decision alone. "If we have a collaborative group of scientists, NIH staff, patient groups, we need to work together to make a decision about what to move forward in this project," Chris said. He asked the parents what they wanted to do, and they threw their support behind cyclodextrin.

At the annual meeting of the National Niemann-Pick Disease Foundation in July 2011, Denny Porter made it official. He told the parents that he aimed to open a cyclodextrin trial.

Chris Hempel didn't attend the meeting, but as soon as she heard the news, she sent an email to Denny. She wrote to him, "I literally almost fainted I am so happy."

10

THE GREATER GOOD

t took over a year of work, but in January 2013, the cyclo-dextrin trial at the NIH was finally a go.

Denny Porter now needed to choose the first three patients to enroll. Although he believed that the drug was safe, once he started giving it to the children, he knew some unexpected, life-altering side effect might emerge. He often reminded his team, and himself, "We could kill a kid."

Enrolling one child in the trial meant another had to wait—wait until the doctors studied the results of those treated first and determined it was safe to keep going, wait until the FDA gave Denny permission to expand the number of open spots or loosen the eligibility rules for participating.

Denny wanted to include very young children in the trial, but the FDA determined that, for the time being, children under the age of seven could not enroll. Denny couldn't be sure how long it might take before the FDA agreed to lower the age requirement. Perhaps six months, maybe a year?

If the drug did turn out to slow down the disease or improve the child's symptoms, waiting to gain access to the compound might mean the difference between a child losing or keeping an essential skill, swallowing food or requiring a feeding tube, walking unassisted or using a wheelchair.

"The choices we are making are not theoretical," Denny said. "They have consequences. And we know the faces that attach to those consequences."

Of the many faces in the NPC community, the one the doctor perhaps knew best belonged to Dillon Papier, the young boy who, along with his mother, had attended the FDA's special advisory hearing a few years earlier determining the regulatory fate of the drug Zavesca.

Dillon was the only child of Mark and Darrile Papier, who lived in Frederick, Maryland, about an hour's drive from the NIH. Dillon had sandy blond hair cut in a pageboy style and twinkling blue eyes. Mark was a high school history teacher and baseball coach; Darrile worked for a mortgage financing company. Dillon had been in and out of the hospital since he was born. Doctors noticed the baby's yellowish skin but told the Papiers it was likely newborn jaundice and would resolve itself. Six weeks later, the jaundice hadn't gone away, and blood tests indicated the baby's liver enzymes were abnormally high. Dillon went back into the hospital for more testing, including a liver biopsy that resulted in a diagnosis of neonatal hepatitis—another misdiagnosis, it turned out.

Other symptoms started emerging. Dillon had trouble crawling and then walking. Doctors knew something was wrong, but they couldn't figure out what it was. In his first three years of life, Dillon had a bone marrow test, two liver biopsies, and, finally, a skin biopsy, as different specialists tried to rule out illnesses and pinpoint what was wrong. Dillon somehow managed to retain his sunny temperament through it all. Going to the hospital, waiting in doctors' offices, and allowing strangers to examine him and draw his blood became as routine for Dillon as the playdates that Darrile organized in the neighborhood. "The nurses and doctors were his friends. Going to the doctor's office was just normal life to him," she said.

The skin culture finally yielded the correct diagnosis, Niemann-Pick disease type C, in 2005, when Dillon was three years old. "We started fundraising quickly," Darrile said. "You feel so out of control when you get a diagnosis like NPC disease." They wanted all the money spent on research to find cures for the disease. At Dillon's nursery school, they ran bake sales and coin drives, activities that by design involved all the children in the class. They created a bulletin board at the school explaining NPC disease, using literature and materials from the National Niemann-Pick Disease Foundation. Darrile soon became an active member of the foundation, serving on the research board that reviewed proposals from scientists seeking grant money for their projects.

The Frederick community also rallied around the Papier family. Parents of children in Dillon's class called Darrile and said their children didn't want presents at their birthday parties. Instead, the children requested donations of money to find a cure for NPC disease. Darrile initially rebuffed the idea; she didn't want the children to resent Dillon or to think they had to give up their presents for him. She didn't want anyone pitying her energetic, exuberant son. "We asked the parents not to do that," Darrile said, "but they told us that their kids insisted." Dillon, with his huge smile and outgoing personality, was a people magnet. He loved baseball and watched his beloved Baltimore Orioles with his father any time a game was televised. He went everywhere with his glove and ball, even to doctors' appointments. When Dillon got a little older and joined the town's Little League baseball team, the other children on the team waited patiently at practice when Dillon got his turn at bat, cheering him on as he slowly made his way to first base. At school, he needed special assistance in the classroom, but despite the difficulties of the disease, Dillon's social skills remained sharp. He remembered the names of all his teachers, the people who served lunch at the cafeteria, and the players on the baseball team his dad coached. Kids gave him high fives as he made his way down the hallway. "He was like the mayor," Mark said about the times Dillon came to visit him at the high school. Dillon exuded joy.

The local newspaper ran an article about Dillon's Army, as Mark and Darrile had taken to calling the growing number of people raising money for NPC research in his name, and the owner of Foster's Grille, a local family restaurant, saw the story and reached out. In 2008, the restaurant started organizing fundraisers on the first Monday of every month. A portion of the proceeds from the Monday nights went to help fund NPC disease research. The designated Mondays turned into a community-wide party and a kind of support group for the Papiers. "It's emotional each month," Darrile said. "You get stuck in your daily routine and feel alone. Then you see the support and it energizes you. You look at everyone who took the time to come here and have dinner and say hello." Different groups of people stopped by; the guys on the baseball team and the friends and fans who always followed in their wake, students in Dillon's classes, parents with kids heading home from after-school activities or music lessons and sports practices. Dillon held court, barely sitting still to eat the two pieces of grilled chicken that the cook knew to prepare whenever the boy came in. Darrile cut the chicken into tiny pieces so Dillon wouldn't choke when he ate—NPC disease could cause swallowing difficulties as the condition progressed—but Dillon often gulped down a handful at a time and had to be reminded to slow down and chew before jumping up to say hello to someone else he spotted entering the restaurant. "Dillon loved it there. He greeted everyone who came in," said Darrile.

Mark and Darrile met Denny Porter a year after Dillon's diagnosis. At the time, Denny was trying to enroll as many patients as possible in his newly minted NPC natural history study. Denny told the Papiers that he hoped the data might help pave the way to an eventual clinical trial. The couple immediately signed up Dillon. They trusted Denny and the NIH and felt fortunate that the nation's leading center of biomedical research was located nearby. From the start, Dillon gravitated toward Denny. Dillon's exuberance and the doctor's rectitude somehow met in the middle. Whenever Dillon arrived at the hospital, he walked down the hallway calling the doctor's name and poking his head in any office with an open door. When Dillon finally arrived at the doctor's office, Dillon always screamed in delight and insisted on giving Denny a hug. "Dillon has insight into people," Darrile said. "He picks people out who are special."

Darrile knew that after the FDA signed off on the Hempel family's compassionate use request, some other parents had also successfully asked the FDA for permission to use the drug in their children. She spoke with Chris and Hugh about their experience with the twins. Darrile and Mark held long conversations about whether they wanted to seek compassionate use permission for Dillon too or to take their chances and wait for an NIH-sponsored cyclodextrin trial to open and, when it did, hope that Dillon was eligible to enroll.

"It is a difficult decision for each family," said Darrile. "At the NIH, we had all the researchers and resources. If we did it on our own, we're not doctors. To me, it is scary. I would have to oversee everything as an advocate, and I am not sure I would understand what I need to do to make sure there is enough oversight."

Mark also worried that any data collected about Dillon in a compassionate use trial wouldn't help other children in the community because compassionate use only involved a single patient and the doctor. "If we go off-site, and if everyone does their own thing, then how do you compare notes?" he asked.

"It isn't a formal study," Darrile added. "We were hoping Dillon participating in a clinical trial would be a stepping-stone for other NPC children to get cyclodextrin." Darrile thought frequently about her frustration and that of the other parents that day at the Zavesca hearing and how later, despite their passionate pleas, the drug ultimately did not win FDA approval. She did not want cyclodextrin to suffer the same fate, with parents and scientists unable to persuade the regulators of a drug's beneficial effects.

THE PAPIERS were not the only parents agonizing over whether to join the trial or seek permission for compassionate use. Daniel Ory, one of the scientists who had helped start the collaborative, often served as a sounding board for the parents. In May, a few months after the NIH launched the cyclodextrin trial, Daniel attended a small gathering set up by one of the parents to attract new donors to fund NPC research. Daniel fielded questions about the disease and his lab's latest experiments. Afterward, the parent confided he was having second thoughts about whether he could wait for his child to be allowed to enroll in the cyclodextrin trial. The parent said he was weighing whether to ask the FDA for permission to give the child the drug through compassionate use. The next day, the parent had arranged to speak with two ethicists he knew for advice, and he asked Daniel to come with him.

They sat together in a small office that opened up on a garden. In the background, children's voices, their laughter, and the chatter of daily life wafted in, along with the warm air. The sounds outside were a constant reminder of how difficult it was to totally separate oneself from the larger world. It wasn't only one child's fate that the parent weighed. In making a decision on behalf of his own child, the parent did not want to harm the other children. In rare disease communities, people knew one another. They met one another's children and spent intense time together. There was a deep bond over the shared fate, the types of challenges that only those immersed in them could truly understand. At family conferences, sometimes parents sat together in a corner, not saying anything, just holding hands or crying. Then there were also the children the parents didn't know, might never meet, but who also seemed to hover in the room. Their voices were like the ones outside, heard in the distance but not seen—children born now but not yet diagnosed with NPC disease, and children who did not yet exist but that would be born in the future.

If he waited for his child's turn to enter the clinical trial, "My child might lose one more level of cognitive ability," he said, adding, "We might not be able to get him back." But if he opted to seek FDA permission to give the drug to the child through compassionate use, he felt he was "choosing my child over the greater good and all these other children."

"Do I have the right to do something that benefits my own child but makes it more difficult for another child?"

The parent proposed a solution: what was needed was a structured way to produce scientific knowledge as a complement to the NIH's formal trial.

The primary goal of scientific research was the creation of generalizable scientific knowledge, the parent said, information that could be used for the benefit of people alive now and future generations not yet born.

With that aim at the forefront, the scientists, parents, and regulators should work together to find a way to do that, whether a child received cyclodextrin in the NIH trial or through a compassionate use request. In diseases as rare as NPC, no patient or patient data should ever be discounted. It was wrong to ask parents to choose between their individual child and the common good—there must be a way for both those aims to be reasonably served.

"We disagree on that," Daniel interjected. If too many patients got the drug through compassionate use, scientists might not be able to enroll the number of people they needed in the trial to prove the drug worked. Without that, the children took on the risks of receiving an untested drug, without the benefit of ever knowing for sure that it worked.

"What an agonizing choice," one of the ethicists said.

The conversation continued, and Daniel stepped outside

to get some air. "Parents should do what they feel is best," he said. "They should be honest and just say, 'We want drugs for our children.' Don't try to rationalize it and say it will help the greater good."

DENNY ENROLLED THE TRIAL'S first patient, a thirteen-year-old girl whose family traveled from Florida to the NIH in order for the child to participate. He told Mark and Dar-rile that Dillon was going to be patient number two. In an effort to try to get as much of the drug as possible into the brain, the doctors chose to deliver the cyclodextrin through a catheter implanted in each patient's brain. The surgery to implant the catheter was routinely performed by surgeons in cancer patients; it was how chemotherapy was often de-livered to people with brain cancer. But there was no getting around the fact that Dillon was going to have to undergo major brain surgery, and the idea scared the Papiers. They discussed the potential risks but still decided to move for-ward. "You have to accept the idea that we are basically human guinea pigs, and that's not easy," Mark said. The couple explained to Dillon what was happening as best they could, but they were never sure how much he under-stood. Dillon didn't ask many questions. "I don't think he understood what the purpose of the trial was," Mark noted.

"He has never questioned why we do fundraising or what Niemann-Pick disease type C is, or even asked what he has. He doesn't ask anything about his condition."

"He just thinks this is normal," Darrile said, and she swept her arm around the hospital room where she was waiting during one of Dillon's many appointments at the NIH, but also in a gesture that seemed to encompass everything about Dillon's life outside the hospital room too. "He visits the dugout of the Orioles and thinks the ballplayers are his friends. He doesn't realize it is unusual to sit with a ballplayer. He watches the players on television and they are the Orioles, but he can go visit them just like he visits Dr. Porter for his appointments. He doesn't see a difference between a huge baseball star and the doctor who treats him or the guys doing the dishes in the restaurant he likes. They're all the same to him. If you're nice, he likes you."

IN EARLY FEBRUARY, Dillon underwent surgery to implant the catheter. Mark and Darrile waited nervously, pacing, for news from the doctors that their son was fine. When a chaplain came by to sit with them, they waved him away. They formed a force field trying to protect their son and could not let their guard down for a moment, even to beseech a deity. The operation went smoothly, the doctors reported to them. Darrile took a breath, then geared up for the next milestone: getting the drug. Nine days after undergoing surgery, Dillon sat with his parents in a small, antiseptic room at the NIH clinical center, waiting for Denny to arrive to oversee the administration of Dillon's first dose of cyclodextrin. The morning of the infusion, Dillon was in an uncharacteristically grumpy mood. His parents had informed him that, as part of the safety procedures surrounding the clinical trial, he wasn't going to be allowed to sleep at home that evening. After Dillon received the drug, doctors wanted to keep him in the hospital for a few days for observation and tests. That meant Dillon and his parents were going to stay at the Children's Inn, a residence for visiting patients and families just across the street from the clinical center, rather than drive home for the night and return to the clinic in the morning for tests, as Dillon preferred. The Children's Inn staff worked hard to make the place as cheerful as possible. They arranged for entertainment for the families, bringing in singers and magicians. There was an air hockey machine in a recreation room, and whenever Dillon stayed in the inn, he challenged Denny to games. But Dillon didn't sleep well when he wasn't at home. Even the prospect of more games of air hockey didn't cheer him up.

The day of Dillon's first infusion, Denny was already worried about the trial, although anyone watching him wouldn't have known. The doctor had a great poker face, smooth and imperturbable. Privately he expressed concern that the first patient to get cyclodextrin in the trial, the thirteen-year-old girl, had developed a bacterial infection. The team didn't believe the infection was due to the drug; cyclodextrin itself appeared safe. But despite the precautions they took when they administered cyclodextrin through the implanted catheter, bacteria grew in the device and caused an infection in the girl. Denny put the girl on a course of antibiotics, but the infection still persisted. Even as they all moved forward with administering the cyclodextrin dose to Dillon, the doctors were debating whether the girl's catheter might have to come out, which would knock her out of the trial.

The infection was a setback, one of the many unexpected things that could sink even a promising, carefully planned clinical trial. Denny was required to report the infection as an adverse event to the hospital institutional review board charged with safeguarding patient safety, as well as to the FDA as part of the standard oversight process in any human trial. It didn't matter that all the specialists involved felt the infection was from the catheter and not caused by the drug itself—anything that harmed a patient could derail the experiment. "If Dillon gets an infection too," Denny said, "they could shut us down."

The care team redoubled all the procedures they were using to keep everything sterile. In the room where Dillon waited, everyone wore two pairs of gloves, not one. They covered their hair and shoes and dressed in scrubs from head to toe. The team wasn't sure if the additional precautions were enough. Among surgeons as experienced as the ones at the NIH, infections almost never occurred. Denny and the other doctors discussed the possibility that the type of bacteria causing the infection, which routinely grows on people's scalps and skin, might be more virulent in people with NPC disease.

That February morning, Denny arrived at Dillon's room, dressed in blue scrubs, his hair covered with a blue cap. Dillon eyed him skeptically and did not offer up his usual smile. "Dr. Porter, I'm mad," Dillon said.

The room felt crowded with the care team and Dillon's parents standing there. Darrile had tried to make the utilitarian quarters feel more festive. Valentine's Day was around the corner, and Dillon's classmates and friends printed well wishes for the boy on cut-out heart-shaped pieces of paper. Darrile hung them on the walls so Dillon could see them.

Denny crouched down on the ground until he was eye-to-eye with Dillon. The boy was dressed in black track pants and a red long-sleeved shirt. "I want to go home," Dillon said.

"Let's play air hockey later," Denny offered.

Dillon was not easily dissuaded. "Why do I have to stay here?" he asked.

"Because we have to watch you," the doctor replied.

Dillon sat with an iPad on his lap. The movie *High School Musical* was playing. Dillon ignored the sight of the cheery actors dancing and singing and didn't turn his attention back to the movie. He seemed disturbed by the poking and prodding going on at the top of his head as the nurses prepared for the infusion. The catheter where the nurses would infuse the cyclodextrin protruded from Dillon's scalp. The nurses inserted a small tube into the catheter and first withdrew some blood for testing. There were six test tubes and plastic syringes lined up on a counter next to Dillon; they planned to draw blood samples through the same catheter before and after Dillon received the cyclodextrin as part of the testing process.

"We get information about you from your blood," one of the nurses explained to Dillon.

A nurse started to clean the opening around the catheter. The hook-shaped stitches the doctors had made in Dillon's skull in order to insert the catheter were still visible. His head was partially shaved where the surgeons had opened up his skull, but his hair was still long everywhere else, giving him an off-beat Mohawk cut. A few drops of the antiseptic liquid dripped into Dillon's eye as the nurses worked, agitating him. Denny took a small cloth and held it to Dillon's eye to take away the sting. "Am I done?" Dillon asked.

"Soon," Denny reassured him. He waited for the boy to settle down again before standing up.

After the blood samples were taken, the nurses prepared to give Dillon the dose of cyclodextrin. The drug was clear and contained in a small vial. The nurse filled the syringe with fifty milligrams of cyclodextrin, the dose the FDA had initially allowed. The amount was lower than what Denny wanted. If all went well with the first patients, Denny hoped to go back to the FDA with a request to increase the dose for future participants. But for now, he needed to prove that he could safely administer the drug.

The nurses put the syringe into the catheter on Dillon's head and told the boy to count to five. "One, two, three, four, five," the boy dutifully called out.

"Starting the medication," the nurse said. Denny marked the time down in a lab notebook and watched the clock. Dillon remained calm while the cyclodextrin was injected. Darrile was now crouched down in front of Dillon, watching her son. While they all waited, Darrile started recounting a story, encouraging Dillon to join in the narration, about a friend from school named Kristina who visited Dillon in the hospital and played air hockey with him. Darrile brought out a photo album and held it up so Dillon and the doctor could both see the pictures. There were photos of Kristina and Dillon baking chocolate chip cookies together, and another of them walking hand in hand down the school hallway delivering the cookies. Darrile recounted how, during a recent air hockey game, Kristina had asked Dillon if she could give him a kiss right in the middle of the game, and when Dillon hadn't objected, she had walked to his side of the table and kissed his cheek.

Dillon finally perked up. He reminded Denny that the doctor had promised to play a game. Dillon boasted that he was going to win.

"I don't use Kristina's technique to win a game," Denny said with a laugh. "Hugs and kisses," Darrile said. Dillon finally relented and offered the adults a small smile. Another nurse watched Dillon's vital signs on a monitor as the drug was administered. Everything looked good, routine.

Around twenty minutes later, the tubes of blood and fluids were filled, ready to go to the lab. The nurses started cleaning everything up. "Bye, Dillon," Denny said. "I'll come by to see you later." Dillon said, "Bye, Dr. Porter." Almost immediately after the others left the room, Dillon turned to his father. "I'm having a meltdown," Dillon told Mark matter-of-factly. There were no tears or yelling, just Dillon's statement. Mark didn't say anything at first, just looked with compassion at his son. Then he found two small disposable cups and poured a thimbleful of juice into each of them. He handed one cup of juice to Dillon and kept the second one for himself. Mark raised his cup and smiled at Dillon. "Cheers," Mark said.

"Cheers," Dillon replied, and smiled back at his father. The two of them touched their plastic cups together, a toast to celebrate the first dose of cyclodextrin. Dillon drained the juice in a single gulp.

11

COMPLICATIONS

C hris and Hugh knew that Addi and Cassi could not enroll in the NIH's cyclodextrin trial. But they still hoped the children's experiences might ultimately help the effort to get FDA approval for the drug. They asked the FDA for permission to deliver the drug through implanted brain catheters, the same way patients in the NIH trial received cyclodextrin. The FDA agreed.

Doctors at the hospital in Oakland, California, surgically implanted the catheters in Addi and Cassi in April 2013. The surgeon told Chris and Hugh that everything went smoothly and that they could take the girls home. Four days after the surgery, the twins were back in Reno recuperating when suddenly Cassi started throwing up.

Chris kept a close vigil by the side of Cassi's bed. The little girl seemed lethargic. When Chris touched her daughter, Cassi's skin felt clammy. Certain that something serious was amiss, Chris called the doctor's office, described Cassi's symptoms, and asked for an appointment.

The nurse told Chris to take Cassi to the emergency room right away. Things moved quickly after that.

Doctors ordered a CAT scan. They looked at the results and immediately called the neurosurgeon at the children's hospital in Oakland who had performed the surgery. Then they came into the room where Chris and Hugh were anxiously waiting and told them the news. Cassi had a brain bleed and had possibly had a stroke. They needed to get her back to the hospital in Oakland—right away. A medical helicopter was on its way. "I was hysterical," Chris said. "They moved Cassi out of the room and intubated her right there."

Chris asked to go with Cassi on the flight, but the pilot refused. The winds were too strong. The pilot worried that any extra weight would make it harder to safely maneuver through the tricky mountain range. Chris watched from the roof of the hospital as the helicopter's engine roared and the medical team whisked Cassi away. "They fired up the helicopter and ran out with her, and she just flew off,"

Chris recalled. Chris wasn't sure she would ever see her daughter alive again.

Chris called her older sister, who lived near Oakland, and asked her to drive right over to the hospital and wait for the helicopter to arrive. Chris's parents were at home watching Addi. Chris and Hugh got in their car and started the four-and-a-half-hour drive. They didn't bother stopping at home to pack. "We just drove," Chris said.

A paramedic called Chris to tell her the helicopter had landed and Cassi was in intensive care. When Chris and Hugh finally arrived at the hospital, the scene in the unit was chaotic. Everywhere Chris looked there were sick children and their families. "There were a lot of people, a lot of noise," she said. A small child lay in a bed nearby, recovering from open-heart surgery. Alarms and buzzers kept going off. Small teams of doctors and nurses raced in and out.

"Cassi was unconscious," Chris said. The surgeon sat with the couple and showed them a picture of Cassi's brain. The image devastated Chris. There was a dark stain around the area where the catheter had been implanted. The doctor explained that the dark spot represented bleeding. Cassi had emergency surgery to remove the blood clot and the catheter. Now they needed to wait for Cassi to wake up. Until she did, her prognosis remained uncertain. Chris and Hugh did not want to leave their daughter's side. A friend of the couple went to their home in Reno, packed a suitcase with clothes, and brought it to Oakland. Cassi regained consciousness twelve days later, but doctors said the little girl needed to remain in intensive care. Chris wasn't sure when they would leave the hospital. The couple started taking turns driving back to Reno so one of them could always be with each of the children.

"You are always second-guessing everything," Chris said one afternoon from Cassi's bedside, while the little girl napped. She worried that Addi might develop a brain bleed too. She called her parents several times a day. "Is Addi acting OK?" she asked them.

The girls' physician let Denny Porter know immediately about Cassi's stroke. Denny sent an email saying he was praying for Addi and Cassi. He asked if the doctors caring for Cassi had any ideas about what might have caused the event.

Chris listed the various theories they threw out. Many people with NPC had low blood platelet levels that could leave them at higher risk for clotting complications after surgery. Perhaps the extreme vomiting Cassi suffered after returning home put pressure on her brain. "There are all kinds of theories at the moment," Chris wrote back to Denny. "Everyone is completely baffled by this."

The weeks in the hospital stretched with no firm timetable about when Cassi might be released. The endless fear and exhaustion ground the couple down.

"It bothers me, the uncertainty, the not knowing about Cassi's prognosis," Chris said. She kept going over the events in the days after the operation. It was like a stone in her shoe that she could not remove. "I don't know why it happened," she said. "You start grasping at everything."

After six long weeks, the couple finally brought Cassi home. She still could not move her left side. Doctors were not sure Cassi would ever regain the ability to move her arm or leg on that side of her body.

Chris and Hugh took turns waking up during the night to turn Cassi so she did not get bedsores. Cassi started to eat some food by mouth again. When Chris asked Cassi to give her a kiss, Cassi opened her mouth and licked her mother. Chris felt grateful for these small gestures. "We could tell Cassi was still there," Chris said.

Chris occasionally experienced flashes from the day. She would be doing routine tasks at home and remember the nausea she felt as Hugh made pinwheel turns on the mountain roads as they sped toward Oakland unsure if their child was still alive. "You feel the anxiety coming on, you can feel it," she said. Chris stopped talking for a moment. "Bad things do happen," she said.

A FEW DAYS after Cassi's stroke, the Papier family hosted their annual fundraiser at the Bowie Baysox game, a minor league team for Dillon's beloved Baltimore Orioles. Dillon threw out the first pitch and spent the entire time running back and forth between the dugout, where he sat with the players, and his friends and family.

After the game was over, Mark, Darrile, and Dillon drove to the Children's Inn across from the NIH's clinical center, where they planned to stay the night. Dillon was due to get his third infusion of cyclodextrin the next morning, on April 15. Darrile had noticed positive changes in Dillon since the little boy started getting cyclodextrin. Even at the low dose, a dose that doctors told them was selected for safety testing and was unlikely to cause any noticeable changes, they saw improvements. Dillon spoke in more complex sentences. At the hospital, Dillon got all the nurses to dance with him to music from the Wiggles, one of his favorite bands. At one point, Dillon jumped high off the floor. The nurse remarked to Darrile she hadn't seen that before; they both attributed his greater dexterity to the cyclodextrin. Delighted by the nurses' excitement, Dillon jumped again and again, entertaining everyone.

For a few days before the third infusion, Dillon experienced low-grade fevers in the evening that broke by the time he woke up in the morning. He continued to go to school, ate normally, and was in good spirits. Darrile said she didn't give the temperature fluctuations much thought because Dillon seemed fine in every other respect. So on the Monday morning of the infusion, the family woke up early at the Children's Inn and walked to the clinical center. Dillon received the infusion and took a nap right afterward. But when he woke up, he told his parents he didn't feel well. He had a fever and threw up. The nurses thought he might have strep throat.

Then things got worse. As part of the trial, some of Dillon's cerebral spinal fluid was drawn after each infusion and tested. Results showed he had an infection. After Dillon threw up, they tested him again. "The numbers were crazy," said Darrile, spiking higher than they had been just a few hours earlier. The doctors worried about the possibility of meningitis. A group of doctors, including infectious disease specialists, met with Darrile and Mark and told them they thought the catheter needed to come out. The idea of another major surgery so soon after the first one frightened the couple, but they agreed to the emergency procedure. The surgeon who had waved goodbye to them a few hours before at the end of his shift, telling them that he was going home to eat a bowl of chili, was called back that same night to perform the procedure. At 11:30 p.m., the nurses wheeled Dillon into the operating room and the surgeon removed the catheter. "We felt disappointed," Darrile said. "But when you are in a clinical trial, you expect the unexpected."

Dillon's and Cassi's experiences weighed on Denny.

When he called the FDA the next day, he explained what happened to the children. For the time being, he said, he was suspending the cyclodextrin trial while the team figured out a way to move forward.

IN THE SUMMER OF 2013, Dana Marella got admitted to the hospital. Her potassium levels were low, and the doctors said they wanted to monitor her for a few days. She seemed to be getting better. Phil and Andrea were optimistic about Dana coming home. But suddenly, her health deteriorated. There was a problem with her kidneys, then her liver. The disease had taken a toll over the years on all her organs. Dana passed away eleven days shy of her twentieth birthday.

The family held a mass at St. Catherine of Siena Church in Riverside, Connecticut. The church was packed. Mourners received a booklet with the order of the service. On the front was a picture of Dana wearing a party hat. She sported bangs and a bright smile. On the back of the pamphlet was a quote: "Our children are a gift, no matter how short a time they are with us."

In his eulogy, Reverend Drew Williams of Trinity Church in Greenwich said that for Phil and Andrea, the family, and also the wider community, "We have to be honest and say this is not the ending we hoped for. This is not what we prayed for. In the pursuit of her healing, Dana's life often felt like a race against time."

Gathered together in the church, the reverend asked the congregation, "We are left with the question—was the race lost? Even the apostle Paul asks—was the race in vain?"

To the reverend, Dana's life represented the power of love. Dana's family and friends recounted how she loved to laugh so hard she dropped to her knees and how much she relished songs from *The Sound of Music*. They had all remembered the day a lady standing in front of them in church turned around and earnestly asked if the Marellas were in fact the von Trapp family.

Dana tried hard to participate in the life around her, even when it was difficult. She went to camp, and the other children were so happy to see her they placed her in a wheelbarrow and raced her around the campsite. When it rained, they all took off their raincoats and covered her so they could continue the game.

The reverend assured the congregation that Dana's illness "is not the final word."

After the service was over, under a blazing sun, family and friends stood in small groups outside the church, comforting one another. Steven Walkley, one of the founders of the collaborative, had grown especially close to the Marellas and drove to the funeral to pay his respects. He looked grief-stricken as he shared words of solace with the family. A parent involved in the collaborative also made his way to Phil and Andrea. He pulled Phil into a tight embrace. The two men sobbed in each other's arms.

ANDREW HAD HIS FIRST SEIZURE about ten days after Dana's funeral. Doctors told them it could be a sign of Andrew's anxiety over his sister's death—or a progression of the disease.

In September, Andrea and her sons were cooking food in the kitchen at a homeless shelter where they regularly volunteered when Andrew had another seizure. "It hadn't happened in weeks," Andrea said.

Soon after arriving home, Andrew had another one. His parents kept him home from school the next day. "I figured we would talk to the doctor and give it a few days," Andrea said.

Six weeks later, the Marella family continued to struggle with Dana's death. There were reminders of the girl's illness throughout the house. A piece of paper remained taped to the wall, listing the medications Dana took starting at 6:00 a.m. through 7:00 p.m. in the evening, when she usually went to bed. Phil had to call the pharmacy to tell them to stop leaving reminders on the answering machine to renew Dana's prescriptions. The hospital bed she used was folded in a corner but hadn't been removed from the home.

Andrew still had not returned to his daily routines, and his parents wondered if they had crossed into a different phase of his disease. A tutor came to the house, but Andrew missed attending classes, seeing friends, and participating in the social stream of school.

"I think our lives have changed no matter what," Andrea said. One day, Andrew did not have seizures, and then he did. Even if Andrew was someday able to return to school, he would need assistance everywhere he went. He might fall unexpectedly and hurt himself. "That is what Niemann-Pick does," she said. "The symptoms change a family's life."

A friend of the family who practiced touch therapy visited the house once a week to work with Andrew. During one visit, Andrew had a seizure while the therapist was there. When the seizure stopped, Andrew looked up and asked her, "Am I going to die from this?"

"Phil and I sat with him and had a pep talk about how well he is doing and how different he is with the disease than Dana was. We did not want him to look at what happened to Dana and think, 'Oh no,'" Andrea said.

"We always maintain that he will be fine," Phil said. "We

are doing great things, and more are on the way. But this is the first time he felt less secure in that assurance."

The warm light of the day streamed into the quiet house. Phil leaned his head closer to Andrea's. "All these families," Andrea said. "We all knew each other, and one by one, we lost them, our children."

12

THE COMMUNITY'S DRUG

Hugh Hempel stood at the podium in the hotel conference room. A surge of nervous energy shot through him. He was used to public speaking, but this was a special audience. Scattered throughout the room were the scientists and parents with whom he had worked, cried, celebrated, and fought for the past six years.

They were all in Baltimore that August in 2013 for the annual meeting of the National Niemann-Pick Disease Foundation. Every year, families traveled to a different city to enjoy a weekend of support and camaraderie amid the constant challenges of living with NPC disease. Activities were planned around the needs of the children. Siblings unaffected by the genetic condition got to attend their own special sessions, talking freely about their lives. Parents chatted and caught up with one another by the side of the pool. The families boarded special buses that ferried them to baseball games or magic shows or other attractions. On the final night, they held a raucous celebration. Parents and children along with doctors and researchers spilled into the center of the dance floor, crying and singing and swaying to the music, their arms wrapped around one another.

Hugh wavered at first about whether he wanted to attend. Cassi was still recuperating from her stroke. She could move her left arm, but not her left leg. Hugh knew he would have to come alone. It was too arduous a journey for Chris and the girls to make with him.

Then Hugh learned the FDA had made an unusual request. Regulators at the agency reached out to the conference organizers and said they planned to attend too. They wanted to meet with the parents and scientists. That was already noteworthy. But they also said they wanted to talk about how to get cyclodextrin approved. Science too often created separations, between researchers and patients, between basic science and translational research, between data collected in a highly controlled setting of a clinical trial and data gathered outside in the real world where patients' and families' lives unfolded. The FDA's presence offered an opportunity to figure out a way to work together. It was an opportunity he couldn't pass up. When the conference organizers asked Hugh to speak at the gathering, he said yes and booked a ticket.

When he looked out at the group, he reminded them and also himself why they were all there. "Sometimes it might not feel like it," Hugh said, "but I can assure each of you that you play an incredibly powerful role in the cyclodextrin story. In fact, none of our dreams regarding cyclodextrin as a treatment for NPC can come true without you."

A large portion of the NPC community participated in clinical research, either at the NIH trial or in compassionate use studies around the country. Hugh knew that the NIH was hoping to find a company to take over the cyclodextrin project and eventually seek FDA drug approval. He asked in his speech that any agreement require the company to also support and move forward the compassionate use program, including the efforts already underway. Cyclodextrin's success was the collective responsibility of everyone in the community, Hugh said. Cyclodextrin was the community's drug.

AFTER THE MORNING'S speeches were over, most of the families and scientists headed to lunch. Hugh hurried over to Andrew Mulberg, then a senior FDA official who was representing the agency at the meeting, and asked for a moment of his time. Hugh wanted to follow up on what the regulator had said at a presentation that morning. If data from the children receiving the drug in the NIH-run trial and data from the children receiving the drug through FDA-sanctioned compassionate use experiments could be collected in a standardized way, the regulator said, the FDA would consider all the evidence when it came time to consider the approval for cyclodextrin.

Hugh said he wanted to ask the regulator if he meant what he said. What needed to be done to ensure that Addi's and Cassi's data, all the children's data, counted in the end?

The value of the compassionate use data had been a source of growing conflict between the scientists and some of the parents, especially the Hempels. The scientists argued that they were stretched thin already. Trying to coordinate the gathering of information about the children taking the drug outside a clinical trial required resources and staff they did not have available, and in their view, it would not sway the FDA anyway when it came time to determine whether to approve the drug. The community's focus, they argued, must be on supporting a clinical trial. Hugh believed in the utility of the compassionate use data, especially given the uncertainties surrounding the FDA approval process. If the results of the trial did not show dramatic benefit, as had happened with the Zavesca trial years before, Hugh argued, the addition of strong compassionate use data might help tip the balance toward an FDA approval. The argument had not gained traction with the scientists, but Andrew's presentation seemed to Hugh to offer a way to bridge the two sides.

Almost as soon as the men started talking, though, Hugh realized that Andrew was not able to go beyond what he had already said. Years later, after Andrew left the FDA, the former regulator and some other colleagues published a paper arguing that given how difficult it was in a rare disease to prove a therapy worked, all the parties involved should pool their data. The paper urged the FDA to give scientists and advocacy groups "top-down guidance" on how to coordinate data collection, even suggesting that Congress get involved and require federal agencies to do more. But Andrew did not offer Hugh such personal opinions or volunteer the FDA's services in brokering a compromise between the parents and the scientists. Instead, the regulator reminded Hugh about the broad challenges involved in drug development and the importance of gathering data in a manner that would enable the regulators to clearly determine if an experimental therapy worked.

Hugh shook Andrew's hand and decided to go join the other parents at lunch. Andrew stopped Hugh at the door. He seemed to want to offer Hugh some kind of encouragement. Questions about outcomes and calculations about risks and benefits could never be fully answered by the scientists alone, Andrew said. "The only way the community can answer them is together."

A few weeks after the conference, the National Niemann-Pick Disease Foundation sent out a message to all the families. The NIH and the FDA had both given their approval for the cyclodextrin trial to start again. Denny and the other researchers planned to deliver cyclodextrin to the children through spinal tap infusions, a frequently used procedure whose inherent safety could be demonstrated by the experiences of Addi and Cassi, both of whom, through their compassionate use program, had each already received around eighty infusions of cyclodextrin in such a manner.

Parents of newly diagnosed children who could not enroll in the NIH trial frequently reached out to Chris and Hugh for advice. The couple and Caroline Hastings, the twins' doctor, shared details about the children's cyclodextrin dosing and regimen, making it easier for other families and doctors to file compassionate use requests.

One of those practitioners, Elizabeth Berry-Kravis, a neurologist at Rush University in Chicago, started out taking care of three patients. Over the years, she received permission from the FDA to oversee the use of cyclodextrin by dozens more, effectively creating the type of large-scale, standardized compassionate use trial Chris and Hugh and some of the other parents had wanted. Liz told the FDA that compassionate use patients offered a unique opportunity to study the drug in the real world. Clinical trials restricted the types of patients who could enroll and had a starting point and an end date. But Liz kept collecting data from patients of all ages and at all stages of the disease's progression, enabling clinicians and scientists to study how the drug changed the trajectory of the disease over the course of years.

When Denny and Liz and other colleagues published a seminal paper about cyclodextrin several years later in the journal *The Lancet*, they shared data from fourteen patients treated in the NIH trial and three patients treated through compassionate use who had all been on the drug for at least a year or longer. The combined results allowed the scientists to conclude that cyclodextrin slowed progression of the disease and was safe to use. The compassionate use data became part of the official scientific record.

After the cyclodextrin trial started again, Phil and Andrea enrolled Andrew. Mark and Darrile brought Dillon back to the NIH for cyclodextrin infusions. Dillon still didn't like staying overnight at the hospital, but Denny's wife, Sherri, always baked chocolate chip cookies and had the doctor bring them by the Children's Inn as a treat for the boy.

Back at home in Reno, Hugh spent more time in his

garden. He continued to expand the backyard, planting more trees and flowers. He liked to see the tree branches drooping with fruit and the riot of color from the flowers. When he was outdoors, he could imagine himself and his family transported to another world, away from the ravages of the disease. He built a pathway that extended around the side of the house and through the garden. Many afternoons, Addi liked to walk up the path, holding on to her parents. When they made it to the top of the hill, they sat on the bench. They looked out at the sweep of the mountains. At that spot, nothing seemed to stand between them and the vastness of the world beyond.

13

LILIES AND DOVES

Denny was working harder than ever as 2015 got underway. One of the main goals set by the parents and the
scientists more than eight years before at the NIH robot lab
had come to fruition. Not only had the community worked
together to identify a promising drug and launch a clinical
trial, there was now a drug company interested in building on their work. The NIH signed a $25 million licensing
deal with a small start-up company, Vtesse. The company
planned to launch an even larger clinical trial in pursuit of
the first FDA-approved drug to treat NPC disease.

The company tapped Denny and Liz Berry-Kravis, the
Rush University doctor, to co-lead the new clinical trial.

The goal was to enroll 51 children that had never been exposed before to cyclodextrin, a daunting task. By the end of 2014, there were more than a dozen people receiving cyclodextrin through compassionate use. Denny was also continuing to collect data on the 14 children who had participated in the NIH-run cyclodextrin trial, people like Andrew Marella and Dillon Papier, who both continued to make monthly treks to the NIH to receive the drug.

Denny stayed at the lab late many evenings, frequently not making it home before 9:00 p.m. He had fewer opportunities to take out the boat and fish. When he had some free time, he liked to work in his backyard. He owned two and a half acres of land, lush and sprawling. When the tree out in the front yard bloomed, it looked like there were iridescent blue lights twinkling on its branches. Denny grew beans and two types of squash, butternut and acorn, but had forgotten to mark which one was which and wasn't sure what was going to come up. There were raspberries and blueberries, tomatoes and cucumbers. Denny dug up roots and got his hands dirty. "It is a kind of therapy," his wife, Sherri, said one sunny afternoon.

Denny worried about the fact that cyclodextrin given at the doses the scientists believed were necessary to slow down the disease also caused hearing loss in the children. Some of the children in the trial were using hearing aids. Then, in February, he got another reminder of the fragility of the children. Dillon remained as social and outgoing as ever, regularly joining his father Mark's weekly poker nights, reveling in the raucous camaraderie of the evenings among the men. But at a recent poker night, Mark noticed something was off. Dillon seemed out of sorts. He threw up at the poker game. Two days later, he woke with a fever and stomach pain. His parents took him to the emergency room, where doctors ran tests and found liver cancer. Dillon underwent surgery so doctors could remove part of his liver. The little boy also needed chemotherapy.

When Denny got the news from Dillon's parents, he was devastated. He kept asking Mark, "How did we miss this?" The cancer diagnosis felt like a gut punch.

Denny went into the freezers at the NIH and retrieved Dillon's frozen blood, to see if there were any clues. He measured the level of alpha-fetoprotein, a protein made in the liver. Healthy people have low levels. Doctors sometimes use the test to help diagnose liver cancer. Denny saw that Dillon's alpha-fetoprotein levels had started to rise two years prior to the liver cancer diagnosis. He wondered if, had he been testing the protein in the children regularly, Dillon's cancer could have been caught earlier. He added alpha-fetoprotein tests for all the children enrolled in the cyclodextrin trial.

The garden offered a place where Denny could assert some sort of order. He pointed to his favorite flowers, the daylilies, whose botanical name means "beauty for a day," because the flowers opened in the morning and died by nightfall. If he saw a connection between his work with children with NPC disease and the daylilies in his garden, he didn't say. The stems of the daylilies often contained over a dozen buds. If gardeners planted and tended them correctly, they could keep flowers blooming all summer long, sometimes stretching into the fall. The colors dazzled when they opened, a riot of velvety maroons, rich purples, yellows the color of lemon drops. The deer loved the flowers too and kept wandering into the Porters' garden to munch on them. Sherri urged her husband to move the daylilies to a different spot, or perhaps to consider planting a different kind of flower, but Denny refused to give up on the daylilies. Sherri said, "He appreciates the blooming flower."

IN JUNE 2016, Chris and Hugh prepared for a four-hour road trip across the mountains to take the girls for the battery of tests required twice a year by the FDA. At twelve years old, Addi and Cassi each weighed ninety pounds, and it was difficult to lift them into and out of the van. Before the trip, Chris painted their nails and did their hair, brushing their ponytails until they were as smooth as sashes. The girls sat on two oversize pink beanbags in the back of the van, propped up on pillows to keep them stable. Chris laid down a pad at the back then cushioned the area with blankets and pillows. Her mother came along too, to help with stretching out the girls' muscles and changing their diapers through the long hours of the trip.

The girls were supposed to be in Oakland for four days, but Chris and Hugh took along supplies to last ten, in case of an emergency. The back of the van was crammed with large plastic buckets containing extra medicine, sippy cups, bibs, diaper wipes, diapers, changes of clothes. They brought a box of trash bags to collect all the dirty laundry. They needed syringes, cotton balls, and rubbing alcohol. They lugged the girls' adaptive strollers. The packing list felt endless. When they finally arrived, it took two hours just to unload.

Addi had a staph infection. Cassi had never recovered full mobility after her stroke and now had difficulty holding up her head. Both girls coughed when drinking water or juice, a sign their swallowing was getting worse. Chris and Hugh pushed the girls in their strollers from room to room, doctor to doctor, sharing the girls' medical journey with each specialist along the way.

Prior to the meeting with the neuropsychologist, Chris sat in the lobby, filling out a questionnaire for each girl designed to assess motor, cognitive, and social skills. Doctors often used the scales to try to identify children with developmental delays who might benefit from early intervention. Chris was brisk, pragmatic, but she seemed weary after the long journey. The questions were a constant reminder of the milestones the girls could not meet, how far they had fallen off the typical path of development. She started reading them aloud. Chris's mother smoothed the girls' hair as they sat in their strollers.

Takes a calm and enjoyable interest in most sights, including colorful or bright things.

"I'm just going to say some of the time," Chris said.

Likes to be swung around, danced with, while in your arms or quickly lifted up in the air.

"If we do that," said Hugh, "they will have a seizure."

You can help your child to calm down.

"They don't get agitated enough to help them calm down," said Chris.

Looks or turns to interesting sounds.

"Half the time," Chris noted.

Chris moved quickly through the checklist. Looks at others' faces when talking. Informs parent when someone comes to the door. She shook her head, crossed out entire sections as she moved along, questions that weren't relevant to the progression of the girls' disease.

"How do we tell doctors they make better eye contact with us? It's our feeling as parents. We try to be realistic about what we see. They aren't moving as well. They aren't swallowing well," she said.

At home, if Chris put M&M's on the table in front of the girls, they knew it was a treat and grabbed for them. They understood their sippy cups went in the mouth for drinking. Most importantly, they held their parents' gaze. Chris valued these interactions most of all because they represented tangible expressions of love; the girls recognized them. She attributed these remaining abilities to the cyclodextrin. "Before they could not look at you," said Chris.

Cassi turned to her mother and reached out an arm, trying to draw her mother's attention. Chris knelt down and brought her face close to Cassi's. "Tell them these are not good questions for me," said Chris. "Tell them I know more than what is on here."

Cassi held her mother's gaze. "Can I have a kiss?" Chris asked her daughter. Cassi nuzzled her mother's cheek and gave her a lick.

DILLON UNDERWENT SURGERY and chemotherapy over the summer. He charmed a whole new set of nurses and doctors, giving them high fives whenever they came to check him. Denny and Sherri visited Dillon in the hospital. Dillon constantly asked the doctors when he could leave and go home to sleep in his own bed. Finally, the doctors told Dillon the day had arrived. Dillon was ecstatic. His hair grew back; he returned to school, reentering the flow of the daily routines he loved. Then, in early 2017, doctors spotted a new shadow in his liver. The cancer had returned.

Mark and Darrile booked a photo shoot for the family for Valentine's Day. Dillon's Make-A-Wish request was to hear a performance of a popular children's band Imagination Movers. The musicians flew in from New Orleans and set up their instruments in the house, with Dillon singing along to all his favorite tunes. When baseball season started, Dillon threw out the first pitch at the home opening game for the Urbana Hawks, the baseball team at the high school where Mark coached the junior varsity team. Dillon called out the nicknames he made up for the boys as they took the field; one of his favorites was a boy Dillon nicknamed "the leprechaun," for the sprightly way the player leaped when he went to catch the ball. Everyone understood that time was running out. The school put up a permanent scoreboard with Dillon's name on it in right field in time for the game. A week after throwing out the pitch, Dillon fell into a coma. He died at the age of fourteen, on April 6, 2017. Dillon was one of 11 children who died of NPC disease in 2017, according to records of community member deaths kept by the National Niemann-Pick Disease Foundation.

The family held a memorial for him at Urbana High School and urged everyone to wear baseball regalia. The players came dressed in their jerseys, with patches on the right sleeves of their uniforms with Dillon's initials on them. Denny and Sherri attended.

OVER THE YEARS, the strain of trying to advance a new model of science while also taking care of seriously ill children took a heavy toll on the community. Chris and Hugh's relationship with some of the scientists and parents in the community had frayed. There were disagreements over the strategic direction of the collaborative. The parents tried to balance their financial support for what they named the "ASAP," or "as soon as possible" project of identifying compounds that could be used right away in the children, with longer-term basic research studies the scientists traditionally pursued. Chris and Hugh felt the scientists had never been comfortable with the ASAP idea, and the couple stopped pooling their money with the other families in order to pursue other efforts with different researchers. Phil Marella and some of the parents who were early members of the collaborative, along with scientists who included NIH's Chris Austin and Denny Porter as well as Daniel Ory and Steven Walkley, coauthored a paper about the model, offering it as a blueprint for other rare disease groups to follow. Chris and Hugh's contributions were acknowledged at the end of the paper, along with those of other early key participants.

The cyclodextrin trial moved forward. Vtesse succeeded in enrolling the patients they needed. In April 2017, Sucampo Pharmaceuticals announced that it had signed a $200 million deal with Vtesse to take over the company and the cyclodextrin trial. Sucampo was so confident about cyclodextrin's potential, and the prospect of FDA approval, that in the press release announcing the deal, they said they expected to launch the drug for sale in 2019.

A month later, Mallinckrodt Pharmaceuticals paid $1.2 billion to acquire Sucampo and its assets. Analysts suggested that the deal gave the company access to Sucampo's already FDA-approved drug treating a form of irritable bowel syndrome and the potential for another drug approval through the NPC cyclodextrin trial, for which results would soon be available.

The interest by the drug companies in cyclodextrin reflected broader changes in the industry. More drug companies were starting to focus their attention on rare diseases after years of patient activism. The FDA said that 17 of the 41 new drugs it approved in 2014 were for rare diseases. At the National Niemann-Pick Disease Foundation's annual conference in 2015, three companies vied at the same time to enroll NPC patients in their drug trials.

So it was a devastating blow for the community when Mallinckrodt announced to investors in November 2018 that the cyclodextrin trial results did not show a clear benefit.

Patients taking cyclodextrin had fared no better when compared to patients in the trial who did not receive the drug. The drug company assured the parents and scientists that they still hoped to find a way forward to FDA approval.

THE PARSEGHIAN FOUNDATION, along with other family groups, decided to hold a community-wide meeting to try to figure out a strategy. Scientists, families, and FDA regulators gathered in a hotel in Hyattsville, Maryland, in March 2019. Chris Hempel found a seat toward the front. She didn't know how she would be greeted, if some of the other parents and scientists would welcome her. Despite the strains of the past years, she wanted to be part of the community effort to support cyclodextrin and other drugs under development.

The meeting itself was a testament to how the model the parents and scientists helped develop had changed the landscape. They had transformed themselves into a community of citizen scientists. Prior to the meeting, families received surveys asking detailed questions about the risks they were willing to take to try experimental drugs and what benefits they felt merited taking those risks. At the meeting, the parents and young adult NPC patients shared their personal experiences living with the disease. They planned to submit a report with all the patient-reported data to the

FDA. They hoped to shape the FDA's thinking as the agency weighed the regulatory fate of cyclodextrin, and examined the data emerging from other drug trials still underway in NPC disease.

The families and scientists had come to believe a one-year trial was not long enough to gather enough data to demonstrate the benefits of cyclodextrin. The disease progressed at different rates in different children. They also wanted the FDA to include the real-world experiences of families like the Hempels, Marellas, and Papiers when making an assessment of the drug's value.

A young mother sitting at the back of the room, her hair hanging past her shoulders, her face still smooth, raised her hand. Her young son with NPC disease had recently suffered serious liver complications, so serious that the doctors felt the boy needed a liver transplant in order to survive. The mother said that in discussing the families' options, the doctors told her that one reason they agreed to the transplant despite the boy's NPC diagnosis was because treatments like cyclodextrin were available, and more were likely on the way. The prospects for this woman's son were better than those Chris and Hugh and Andrea and Phil and Darrile and Mark and earlier generations of parents faced when their own children were diagnosed. The woman's voice quavered when she told the group that she wanted to thank all the patients and parents who had come before, those whose sacrifices and work made it possible for her family to have more options. She clung to the belief that the medicines they helped advance might keep her son healthy enough to live to see the next medicine.

This was the closest the community had come to crafting a narrative not just where all their perspectives could exist, but that carried equal authority with those of the scientists. And although not all the parents with younger children knew every detail, those gathered that day understood the larger message: the future looked different because other families, citizen scientists, clinicians, and researchers had worked to make it so.

During the break, one of the parents who met and worked with Chris in the earliest days of the collaborative approached her. They hadn't spoken in a long time and greeted each other awkwardly; it was hard to find the words. When the parent came over, he handed Chris a can of Diet Dr Pepper. Years before, when they had first started out, Chris loved to drink Dr Pepper. During all the long meetings with the scientists, she fueled herself on it. Now she no longer drank soda. She hadn't had a Dr Pepper in years. She looked at the can, uncertain if she should tell him. At first, she saw the drink as a sign of how they didn't really know each other anymore, how different things were now, in large important ways and this smaller one too. But then Chris saw the drink for what it was, a quiet gesture, a measure of recognition from one parent to another of all they had accomplished. She realized how much the offer meant to her. She cracked open the can and took a sip.

THE MORNING OF JULY 4, Chris and Hugh noticed that the girls were having more difficulty breathing. Hugh called the girls' doctor, who told them to take the twins to the hospital. Tests revealed that Addi and Cassi had human parainfluenza virus, a common pathogen that caused upper and lower respiratory infections, such as pneumonia. The girls were given oxygen support and sent to the intensive care unit. The hospital allowed the children to share a single room on the unit. At first, Chris and Hugh thought the latest emergency would end the way others had, that after a few days the girls' situation would stabilize and they could all go home together, just as they had in the past. But years of damage from NPC had taken a toll. Their muscles and lungs were weak; they had trouble coughing and continued difficulty breathing. Chris and Hugh held the girls and told them how much they loved them. A few hours later, the children passed away, first Addi, then, twenty minutes later, Cassi. So many times, Chris said, she cried thinking that death might separate the girls from each other. But just as they had come into the world together, that was how they left it.

A few months later, on a beautiful September day, the Hempels held a celebration of life at their home in Reno. The girls' bedroom overflowed with mementos of their lives together. When the girls were first born, Chris created memory boxes, two sets, consisting of three round boxes stacked one on top of the other. Over the years, she squirreled away items in them—locks of hair, the first tooth, the first shoes, a note to Santa Claus asking for a dollhouse.

On the girls' bed, Chris arranged clothes and toys that represented the stages of the girls' lives. Everything was grouped in twos. Two pink stuffed bunnies, with two baby dolls sitting in their laps. Two bottles, pacifiers, and infant onesies, each emblazoned with the words "Perfect Pair." Two tote bags hanging from the knobs of the bedpost, one with a "C" on the front, the other with an "A." Two tiny pairs of patent leather pink baby shoes.

Chris worked for weeks, sorting through their clothes. The dresses from their fifteenth birthday party, the last one they held, hung above the windows, and the light from outside illuminated the intricate pattern of the sequined bodices. Other frocks they wore over the years were still hanging inside the closets. Chris gave some of the dresses away and planned to make quilts from other clothes to give to family members.

The house overflowed with family and friends; scientists, doctors, other NPC parents, parents of children with different rare diseases who had reached out to learn from the Hempels' experiences. In the months since the girls died, Hugh had let the backyard grow wild. Many of the plants and flowers had not been cut back; they spilled everywhere, like Hugh's grief. He could not bring himself to tend the garden, not yet.

Over the years, Hugh had created outside a place of refuge for the family, their own Eden. He took pieces of old chairs and brass tubes, broke them apart, and set them against a back wall; plants and vines grew amid them, a mixture of the modern world and the bucolic, the machine amid the garden.

Peaches hung heavily from the trees, about to drop to the ground. Raised wood boxes contained tomato plants, cherry and beefsteak. Flowers and blooms were everywhere. Along the carved path where Chris and Hugh frequently took the girls, a wooden table stood, a large slab upon which a feast might be served.

Chris and Hugh asked the guests to gather under the tent at the back of the house. There were many people they wanted to honor and thank. The doctors and nurses who took care of the girls, scientists who worked on the cyclodextrin project, caregivers who arrived in shifts and became members of the family, a special education teacher who practiced every morning with the girls on the computer. Chris cried throughout the morning; seeing old friends, acquaintances, all the people who were part of Addi's and Cassi's lives walking through the house, she broke down.

Hugh addressed the crowd with a microphone, explaining that they wanted a way to remember the girls and to honor the community that loved and sustained them. Hugh asked Chris to hold up a birdcage. Each cage contained two white doves—twins, said Hugh. They were homing pigeons bred for their ability to travel long distances. Family, friends, caregivers, teachers, and doctors were invited to come forward, open a cage, and release the birds. The grief came in waves.

When Addi and Cassi's teacher opened the cage door, the doves did not immediately fly away. One bird perched on the edge, almost as if it wanted to stay a little longer and could not bear to leave those gathered there. But then the doves took flight, they flew away, first one, then the other. Everyone looked up at the sky. The light and the glare of the day was bright, the sky glistening. It was hard to track the course of the birds. They were there, and then they were gone, flying into the light above.

14

THE CATHEDRAL
OF SCIENCE

During my bioethics studies, one of the professors assigned us to read the short story "Cathedral," written by Raymond Carver. At first, I wasn't sure why. In class, we were often presented with examples of people confronting real-life medical problems and asked to talk about the ethical tensions. The cases almost always involved people making difficult moral choices based on limited information and acting under tremendous emotional stress—doctors trying to decide how to allocate scarce and urgently needed medicines or interventions and families divided among themselves about whether an incapacitated loved one might choose to move forward with a risky procedure whose out-come was uncertain. "Cathedral" did not describe such situations. Instead, it was ostensibly a quiet story about a couple whose marriage seemed to be unraveling. The couple was down on their luck. They were still together, sharing their daily lives and their home, but they seemed distant from each other. They didn't talk much or seem affectionate. They lacked insight into each other's motivations, hurts, sorrows, and aspirations. Despite their physical proximity, the contours of each other's interior lives remained hidden and opaque.

The woman invited an old friend, a man who was blind and whose wife had just died, to come and stay with them. The narrator was curious about the man, especially because he shared a history with the woman. But he was also un-settled by the blind man's presence and the hold he appeared to have on the woman's emotions. This sensation of discomfort grew throughout the visit, as the narrator real-ized how their guest, through careful and attentive listen-ing, was far more attuned to the woman than he was. The blind man, he came to understand, saw the woman more clearly than her husband did.

I thought a lot about this story and how it related to the collaborations that I witnessed the scientists and patients and families struggling to build. Like the married couple in the story, the participants shared the same space and developed an intimacy that grew when people were witnesses to others' pain. But many times, despite their efforts, they still didn't see one another clearly. They ascribed motivations to the others' actions that pushed them apart. And even when they tried to do things differently, to truly act as full partners, the scientists largely remained in the seat of power due to the way the entire edifice had been built.

At one point in "Cathedral," the woman said she was going to sleep, leaving the men together in an awkward silence. They didn't quite know how to communicate, or what they might share in common outside the woman's presence. The narrator turned on the television and started to watch a show about the building of a cathedral. He asked his guest, "Do you have any idea what a cathedral is? What they look like, that is? Do you follow me? If somebody says cathedral to you, do you have any notion what they're talking about?"

The narrator proceeded to try to describe a cathedral but found that his words were inadequate. He struggled to convey what a cathedral looked like to someone who had not seen one for himself. They were tall, the man offered. They were made of stone, he added. Finally, his guest suggested that instead of talking about the cathedral, they collaborate and draw one together. The narrator retrieved some pens and paper, and the blind man put his hand over his host's hand. They drew the shape of a cathedral. You initially thought that the narrator was the one who would determine in the end how the cathedral would look; he was the only one who had seen one, so he should have been the authority. But actually, at the end of the story, it was the blind man who realized the most important element that was missing from the picture. "Put some people in there now," the man said. "What's a cathedral without people?"

THE HISTORY OF MODERN SCIENCE has been shaped by the separation of citizens from scientists. The cleaving originated in the understandable desire to create a profession. Scientists developed professional guidelines and established academic programs where people could acquire the necessary skills and the credentials that went along with them. But the effort eventually went too far. Scientists set themselves apart from the issues that were most urgent to patients struggling to find treatments and answers today. They essentially built a cathedral without people in it.

In recent years, scientists have paid more attention to public engagement, especially surrounding controversial scientific advances such as the development of drugs that treat diseases by editing people's DNA. But even these efforts often fail to put patients at the center. Researchers at the University of California, Berkeley, conducted in-depth interviews with scientists who use gene editing in their research, asking them questions about how their work might affect the lives of people who have lethal genetic diseases. The scientists enthusiastically discussed their latest advances and the prospect for finding cures, the paper's authors noted, but showed "much less apparent interest in discussing the complex and diverse needs of people with diseases." Jodi Halpern, a professor of bioethics and medical humanities at the university, and one of the study's authors, told me that scientists learn about professional ethics such as sharing credit and authorship of papers and the importance of proper data management but do not get sufficient training around an equally crucial topic: "What will your decision-making mean for people living with the disease?"

As a result, patients' priorities are not always taken into account when important choices are made about what drug to study, what trial to design, what research to fund. Patients who want to do their own research do not have access to the infrastructure and tools that they need. When patients organize themselves and succeed in collecting data, they can find it difficult to disseminate their findings within the professional science journals, a crucial step in persuading doctors and others to eventually adopt new knowledge and change existing clinical practices.

Too often, the burden and responsibility for being recognized as equal partners falls more on patients and their families than on scientists. Patients who want to be taken seriously know they must learn how to speak the language of the researchers. They figure out a way to fit their research questions into the scientists' existing agenda, rather than the scientists trying to adapt their work to what patients consider most urgent.

THE NPC FAMILIES DEMONSTRATED that motivated patients and advocates can create science. Chris Hempel, someone who did not think much about the scientific process before her children were diagnosed with NPC disease, started reading about advances in fields outside NPC disease. She forged connections with scientists even beyond the NPC disease community. In one instance, she came across an article in a journal by scientists proposing that cholesterol crystals that form in arteries might trigger inflammation and drive heart disease. It got her thinking that the cyclodextrin compound her twins were taking might also help dissolve the cholesterol crystals in patients suffering from heart disease. She shared her hypothesis with the lead scientist, who worked with her to test the idea, eventually publishing a paper of which Chris was a coauthor. She also flew to the prestigious Karolinska Institute in Stockholm, the cathedral of science where the Nobel Prizes are awarded every year, at the invitation of scientists there who wanted to learn about the community's efforts to develop cyclodextrin.

Phil Marella, along with other parents and professional scientists, continues to work together to try to identify promising drugs to treat NPC disease. They have advised families with children suffering from other disorders about how to create a research collaborative that is open to both citizen scientists and professional scientists.

And when Mallinckrodt announced in January 2021 that the company was shuttering the cyclodextrin program, the parents and scientists refused to abandon it. They urged the FDA to weigh patients' lived experiences and started working with a new company that in May 2021 bought the rights to the drug. They still hope to get FDA approval for the compound they found and developed together. There is no guarantee they will ultimately succeed, of course. But in an August 2021 letter to the FDA following a community "listening session" with the agency, the parents insisted on recognition of the value of the data generated by the community, reminding the regulators, "you indicated that parents are the experts."

EFFY VAYENA, a professor of bioethics at the Swiss Federal Institute of Technology and one of my advisers during my master's program, has pushed for the creation of a new social contract to help support collaboration between scientists and citizen scientists. There are already well-established ethical principles for research involving human subjects such as the Nuremberg Code, which was adopted following horrific experiments conducted on people by the Nazis during World War II. Other requirements got added over the ensuing decades by hospitals and universities. Scientists today must obtain ethical and other reviews before their institutions and regulators will allow them to start enrolling patients in trials. But the current rules are not designed to address issues raised by experiments run by and with patients.

In a meeting held in London, Effy and other scientists and researchers tried to hammer out a version of a new contract that also addressed the ethics of patient-led research. The starting place of the meeting was the notion that people who are not professionally trained scientists can generate important knowledge. The participants in the meeting wanted a document that recognized that both citizens and scientists had responsibilities toward society, and toward one another, to produce work that could benefit everyone. It was not enough for scientists to tell patients and citizen researchers that they didn't produce rigorous science; professional scientists had an obligation to help the citizen scientists do better work. Parents may fund and drive scientific projects to save the lives of their own children, but the experiments could be designed and data collected in ways that would also benefit the wider community.

When setting out to work together, citizen and professional scientists don't always think about writing a social contract or a declaration of common principles such as a constitution. Parents who learn their children have a fatal disease are overwhelmed by the diagnosis. They must balance the pursuit of science with caregiving of seriously ill children and healthy siblings. Many times, one parent must quit a job in order to take on the burden of navigating the healthcare system, causing huge financial strains on a family's resources. Professional scientists have their own set of pressures. In order to secure funding for their labs or tenure at their universities, they must produce a steady stream of papers. They are familiar with existing ethical and regulatory frameworks but may not be eager to sit down with citizen scientist partners to devise a whole new set of rules. Recognizing such limitations, the London group proposed ways to facilitate such collaborations, including creating a web-based platform where research projects could be registered and followed and developing online tools that anyone could download that included checklists and potential obstacles that could be discussed at the outset. Chris Austin, the former NIH scientist whose lab hosted the first meeting of the collaborative, said he regretted that the group didn't try to establish a guiding framework at that first meeting, or in the many meetings that came afterward. Such a set of guidelines might have helped resolve disputes that inevitably arose over the years, he said, and provided benchmarks to better assess the value of the work they did. "Having a conversation and writing it down is worth doing," Chris said to me in a recent conversation after he left the government to become the CEO of a drug company called Vesalius Therapeutics. "When you try to create a new paradigm, you run smack into all the old paradigms while doing it."

THE GOVERNMENT has an important role to play in ensuring the future of collaboration between professional scientists and citizen scientists and a vested interest in helping these partnerships succeed. The FDA stated in its 2016 "Guidance for Industry" report that the primary purpose of compassionate use programs is to "diagnose, monitor, or treat a patient's disease or condition rather than to obtain the kind of information about the drug that is generally derived from clinical trials." But what if the FDA, in conjunction with the wider scientific and patient community and under certain conditions, took a more expansive view?

In many cases, if a patient is truly weeks or months away

from death, there may simply be no time to do anything other than to give early access to an experimental therapy through compassionate use and hope for the best. But there are many neurodegenerative diseases, such as the motor neuron disease ALS or NPC disease, where quality-of-life declines but patients can survive for years. It is a tremendous loss for science to let data generated outside clinical trials go to waste.

When doctors and families apply for compassionate use access in such cases, FDA scientists should work closely with them to determine or insist on standardized health outcomes and information that will be measured each time the drug is taken. When subsequent clinicians then apply for compassionate use permission, they should be provided with the same forms. The collection of standardized data should be a condition of the FDA signing off on company-sponsored trials as well.

The FDA has an important role to play in instructing citizen scientists on how to go about collecting compassionate use data on their own. Putting patients at the center of science should not be limited to inviting one or two patients at a time to sit on a committee or attend a meeting. It should also entail helping citizen scientists to gather data in ways that will advance scientific knowledge. The FDA should create new channels to engage citizen scientists. FDA staff members knowledgeable about citizen science should be officially tasked with addressing any questions and provide immediate feedback on proposed studies. Citizen scientists trying to develop drugs should be allowed to request the same type of meetings the FDA already holds with scientists and with companies, offering insights and feedback on proposals to start clinical trials. The NIH should help citizen scientists find the kind of expertise they need to move their projects forward, and integrate patients into partnerships from the conception of the idea, not after the rules of engagement have already been worked out.

WE NOW STAND at a pivotal moment in the field of science. The Covid-19 pandemic has presented an opportunity to make systemic change. A group of patients still suffering symptoms months after falling ill decided to take matters into their own hands and self-organize. They, and not professional scientists, gave the syndrome a name: Long Covid. "The fact that Long Covid was collectively made, identified, and named by patients is a crucial moment in medical history," Elisa Perego, a Covid patient who helped name the disease, told me.

Long Covid advocates built on the work of communities that came before them like the NPC families. Covid patients met one another online and formed patient-led research groups. One group, called the Patient-Led Research Collaborative, created a detailed survey that resulted in a valuable portrait of the Long Covid sufferer. They posted their results online before the traditional research apparatus could even get going or fully recognized that mild or moderate cases of Covid could lead patients to suffer from long-term complications. The then NIH director Francis Collins cited the citizen scientists' work, including key findings in his blog and steering people to the group's website. Leaders of the patient-led research group wrote a formal scientific paper, which they posted on the same public website used by scientists during the pandemic to rapidly disseminate new information about Covid.

Some of these advances were made possible because Covid-19 was caused by a new virus without recognized or established experts. During the outbreak of Covid, things that used to take years to accomplish happened rapidly— the sharing of gene sequences of the virus, the creation of diagnostic tests, the development and then rollout of vaccines. Innovative models for developing drugs sprung up, as well as collaborations between patients and researchers.

Science should not return to the old ways. Chris Austin says he frequently gives speeches about the opportunity presented by Covid to change the way science is done.

"If we are willing to accelerate the process for Covid

patients but we are not willing to do it for cancer or Alzheimer's or rare disease patients, then we are explicitly saying the lives of patients with Covid are more important than the lives of rare disease patients," Chris said. "If you are willing to live with that, then fine, but I imagine most of us are not. Covid showed us that we can make changes happen."

The Patient-Led Research Collaborative will now have an opportunity to test some of their ideas, announcing in April 2022 that they received $3 million from the Balvi fund, which was set up by a cryptocurrency pioneer to support Covid research that is often overlooked by traditional funders. Scientists are the ones who usually decide what hypotheses should be tested, typically building on questions that they have studied before, said Hannah Wei, a Long Covid patient and one of the founders of the collaborative. The Long Covid group is instead planning to test patient-generated hypotheses that grow out of their experiences with the disease. One of the first projects the group is tackling addresses concerns raised in online forums by people worried about what will happen to them if they get infected again. "We need information that is useful for us now," Hannah said.

Helen Burstin, a doctor who is CEO of a coalition of medical specialty societies that is also collaborating with the Long Covid group, says in order to make further gains, citizen scientists need access to the same resources that sustain professional scientists, including the opportunity to embed themselves in labs and seek research funding. "The patient-led research model is extraordinary but it is a heavy lift for many patients," Helen told me. "They need institutional support from the research community to support them. The next step is finding a way to build bridges between patient-led research and what is already happening in the broader research community. We want to bring citizen science into the traditional research community but not take it over."

IT TAKES TIME for the formal infrastructure of modern science to get up and running, whether during a pandemic or when a group of parents sit around a table with scientists in an NIH lab and decide they want to work together as partners to find a drug. The opportunity to collect data must start right away and not wait until the system rattles to life. By the time formal studies get going, and the professionals and institutions and review boards all sign off, tremendous amounts of information could be lost. Every scrap of data is vital for helping figure out what questions to ask next and how to direct resources and identify the most urgent issues.

Working together, science can realize its fullest potential—generating useful, beneficial information that improves the lives of patients today and provides direction for the patients of tomorrow.

Matt Might, whose son Bertrand died in 2020 from a rare disease, published a document online that he calls "The Algorithm for Precision Medicine." He wanted to help other parents and patients in the future, gathering in one place all the things he and his fellow citizen scientists learned. Matt wrote in the introduction to the document that, despite his son's death, he planned to continue updating the information. He called the work "a living document," adding, "In a real sense, this document will never be finished, so please check back." Matt's words are a reminder that the task of improving science falls on all of us.

When I think about the work the NPC community did, and the efforts of all the citizen scientists I have met over the years, I am reminded of that Raymond Carver story. They built a collaboration through their own sacrifices—the families first and foremost, but also the scientists, the doctors, the government officials, and many others who realized that something wasn't working and joined the families in trying to find a better way. They wrote papers, organized meetings, and shared their experiences with other groups. They kept going in order to benefit the next generation of children, some of them even after their own children had died. They helped drive a larger movement—and their model, despite any imperfections or flaws, inspired many other patients along the way. Most importantly, they kept asking the question that still demands an answer: What is a cathedral unless there are people in it?

ACKNOWLEDGMENTS

Writing a book shares something important in common with the practice of science: Both benefit from the help of collaborators.

I'm grateful to the many people in my community who supported me and whose thoughtful suggestions helped improve my work.

Many thanks to the Robert Wood Johnson Foundation for reaching outside the world of academia and granting a newspaper reporter an Investigator Award in Health Policy Research. The grant allowed me to launch the reporting that eventually led to this book.

The Wall Street Journal has been my professional home for

more than two decades, and I am fortunate to work with many generous, dedicated, and talented colleagues. My profound thanks to the paper's editor in chief, Matt Murray, and the health and science coverage chief, Stefanie Ilgenfritz, for their steadfast support of this project over the years. Sam Enriquez deftly edited the series I wrote about the early years of the collaborative that was published by the *Journal*.

The Jonathan Logan Family Foundation and the Logan Nonfiction Program at the Carey Institute for Global Good offered me a place to write and think, not to mention the camaraderie of an inspiring group of people. Carly Willsie and Josh Friedman nurtured the special community that formed there. I'm grateful for the feedback on early chapters of the book from the autumn 2018 fellows, and the continued advice and friendship of Susan Berfield and Meg Kissinger after we all returned home.

Rebecca Brendel, Christine Mitchell, and Bob Truog opened the doors of Harvard Medical School's Center for Bioethics to me and offered important feedback on my ideas. Effy Vayena, my faculty adviser turned dear friend, has done path-breaking work on the ethics of patient-led research. She was generous enough to read and critique chapters of the book. A paper she coauthored with John Tasioulas, called "'We the Scientists': A Human Right to Citizen Science," helped inspire the title of this book.

Martha Montello, whose narrative bioethics class led me to read Raymond Carver's fiction with fresh eyes, has continued to steer my thinking in new directions. I am grateful for her friendship and wise counsel. Many thanks as well to Diana Alame, Ha Jung Lee, and John Limouze, fellow members of Martha's bioethics writing group, who were considerate, generous readers of several chapters. Toby Lester and Mark Kramer, both graceful writers of narrative nonfiction, made valuable editing suggestions on an early draft.

My agent, David Doerrer, believed the story of a collaboration between families and scientists could shed light on the broader problems of modern science. Courtney Young, my gifted editor at Riverhead Books, shaped and improved the book in every possible way and was an invaluable sounding board throughout the entire process.

Many scientists generously took time to meet and speak with me. While not all of them are named in the book, their help made a difference. Special thanks to Chris Austin, Caroline Hastings, Benny Liu, Daniel Ory, Marc Patterson, Denny Porter, and Steven Walkley, who answered all my many questions. I respect their commitment to the ideal that public engagement is part of the duties of a scientist.

Words are not adequate to express my appreciation to the many members of the NPC community who spoke with me over the years. Some did not want their names in the book, and I want to recognize the significance of their contributions here. I am humbled by the generosity of the Hempel, Marella, and Papier families, who allowed me to spend time with their wonderful children and to chronicle the most profound and private moments in their lives. I hope the memories of Addi, Cassi, Dana, and Dillon comfort and inspire them.

ACKNOWLEDGMENTS

My love and gratitude to my father, Bob Dockser, for his unwavering support, and to Judy, Lynne, Richard, and Sam for buoying my spirits along the way. And to Ronen, Eden, and Yuval, you are my heart—and my favorite collaborators of all.

NOTES

INTRODUCTION: WE THE SCIENTISTS

I drew on a growing and excellent literature describing the history, contributions, and significance of citizen science. Steven Epstein's seminal work about the HIV/AIDS advocacy movement, *Impure Science: AIDS, Activism and the Politics of Knowledge*, continues to influence my thinking. The paper "Embodied Health Movements: New Approaches to Social Movements in Health," published in the journal *Sociology of Health & Illness* by a team of researchers led by the sociologist Phil Brown, demonstrates how the reach of health activists can extend beyond their own disease as other patients draw inspiration from their work. Rebecca Dresser's books *When Science Offers Salvation: Patient Advocacy and Research Ethics* and *Silent Partners: Human Subjects and Research Ethics* offer compelling accounts of the emergence and growing power of patient advocates, the challenges they pose to the research establishment, and how they can become recognized as experts. I also benefited from Darlene Cavalier and Eric B. Kennedy's excellent collection of essays, *The Rightful Place of Science: Citizen Science*, and Caren Cooper's fascinating account of the birth of the movement in her book *Citizen Science: How Ordinary People Are Changing the Face of Discovery*.

xiii **As a reporter:** The Pulitzer Prizes, "The 2005 Pulitzer Prize Winner in Beat Reporting," Pulitzer.org, accessed March 7, 2022, www.pulitzer.org/winners/amy-dockser-marcus.

xiv **Doctors diagnosed metastatic:** American Cancer Society, "Cancer Statistics Center," accessed March 7, 2022, https://cancersta tisticscenter.cancer.org/#!.

xiv **Even if they:** "Orphan Drugs Continue to Struggle During Approval Process," The Association of Clinical Research Professionals (blog), May 14, 2018, https://acrpnet.org/2018/05/14/orphan -drugs-continue-struggle-approval-process.

xv **My mother died:** Amy Dockser Marcus, "A Cry in the Dark: When a Rare Cancer Strikes, a Patient Has Few Places to Turn," *The Wall Street Journal*, March 20, 2006, https://www.wsj.com /articles/SB114235179275597797.

xvii **One study I read:** Mette B. Steffensen, Christina L. Matzen, and Sarah Wadmann, "Patient Participation in Priority Setting: Co-Existing Participant Roles," *Social Science & Medicine* 294 (February 2022): 114713, https://doi.org/10.1016/j.socscimed .2022.114713.

xix **These people called themselves:** Amy Dockser Marcus, "Citizen Scientists," *The Wall Street Journal*, December 3, 2011, https:// www.wsj.com/articles/SB10001424052970204621904577014330551132036.

xxi **Until the late nineteenth:** Laura J. Snyder, *The Philosophical Breakfast Club: Four Remarkable Friends Who Transformed Science and Changed the World* (New York: Broadway Books, 2011).

xxiii **The data could:** Susan Leigh Star and James R. Griesemer, "Institutional Ecology, 'Translations' and Boundary Objects: Amateurs and Professionals in Berkeley's Museum of Vertebrate Zoology, 1907–39," *Social Studies of Science* 19, no. 3 (August 1989): 387–420, http://www.jstor.org/stable/285080.

xxiii **But the standardization:** Star and Griesemer, "Institutional Ecology," 407.

xxiii **"The creation of new":** Star and Griesemer, "Institutional Ecology," 388.

xxv **The people who wrote:** Effy Vayena and Josh Tasioulas, "Adapting Standards: Ethical Oversight of Participant-Led Health Research," *PLOS Medicine*, March 12, 2013, https://doi.org/10.1371/journal.pmed.1001402.

xxvi **So began what:** Amy Dockser Marcus, "Trials: A Desperate Fight to Save Kids & Change Science," *The Wall Street Journal*. November 14, 2013, http://graphics.wsj.com/trials/#chapter=1.

xxix **They even gave:** Felicity Callard and Elisa Perego, "How and Why Patients Made Long Covid," *Social Science & Medicine* 268 (January 2021): 113426, https://doi.org/10.1016/j.socscimed.2020.113426.

xxix **and found themselves cited:** Francis Collins, "Citizen Scientists Take on the Challenge of Long-Haul COVID-19," *NIH Director's Blog* (blog), September 3, 2020, https:/directorsblog.nih.gov/2020/09/03/citizen-scientists-take-on-the-challenge-of-long-haul-covid-19.

1. THE HERE AND NOW

This chapter is based on author interviews with Chris and Hugh Hempel, including on June 8, 2009; November 9, 2009; February 20, 2010; and March 2, 2013, and interviews with the couple's friends and colleagues Donna Burke, Catherine Corre, Carol Leveroni, James Messemer, and Rosanne Siino.

2 **They had clear:** Quotes and descriptions of the children's development are from the baby books that Chris Hempel kept. She shared them with the author.

11 **In his expert:** Marc Patterson's notes describing his findings from Addi and Cassi's visit were shared with the author by Chris and Hugh Hempel.

18 **Yet by the time Addi:** "NIH Scientists Identify Gene for Fatal Childhood Disorder, Niemann-Pick Type C," National Human Genome Research Institute, July 1997, https://www.genome.gov/10000889/1997-news-release-niemannpick-type-c-gene.

2. A DIFFERENT FEAR

This chapter is based on author interviews with Phil and Andrea Marella, including on April 5, 2013; October 9, 2013; and October 31, 2013.

28 **After Dana's diagnosis:** Dana's Angels Research Trust, accessed March 15, 2022, https://danasangels.org.

3. THE FISHING EXPEDITION

This chapter is based on author interviews with Denny and Sherri Porter, including on July 9, 2009; April 20, 2009; December 9, 2009; July 6, 2016; and June 26, 2017. The author visited the Porters at home in June 2016.

37 **In a paper Denny:** Elaine Tierney et al., "Analysis of Short-term Behavioral Effects of Dietary Cholesterol Supplementation in Smith-Lemli-Opitz Syndrome," *American Journal of Medical Genetics Part A* 152A, no. 1 (January 2010): 91–95, https://doi.org/10.1002/ajmg.a.33148.

4. THE CATALYSTS

Descriptions of the trip to Brazil are based on author interviews with Daniel Ory, Marc Patterson, and Steven Walkley in March 2013. The scientists and parent shared with the author their email correspondence and the document they wrote together in preparation for the trip.

48 **The trial failed:** M. C. Patterson et al., "The Effect of Cholesterol-Lowering Agents on Hepatic and Plasma Cholesterol in Niemann-Pick Disease Type C," *Neurology* 43, no. 1 (January 1993): 61–64, https://doi.org/10.1212/wnl.43.1_part_1.61.

52 **A Michigan scientist:** Thomas A. Finholt, "Collaboratories," *Annual Review of Information Science and Technology* 36, no. 1 (February 2005): 73–107, https://doi.org/10.1002/aris.1440360103.

5. THE OPERA SINGER

This chapter is based on author interviews with Chris Austin, including on February 9, 2012; April 12, 2013; May 2, 2013; May 29, 2013; and June 18, 2013.

58 **For that paper:** C. P. Austin and C. L. Cepko, "Cellular Migration Patterns in the Developing Mouse Cerebral Cortex," *Development* 110, no. 3 (November 1990): 713–32, https://doi.org/10.1242/dev.110.3.713.

65 **The mother was:** Maria Eriksson et al., "Recurrent *de novo* Point Mutations in Lamin A Cause Hutchinson-Gilford Progeria Syndrome," *Nature* 423 (May 2003): 293–98, https://doi.org/10.1038/nature01629.

6. THE BROAD JUMP

For the history of cyclodextrin, I drew on interviews with Benny Liu, József Szejtli, Steven Walkley, and Cristin Davidson. József Szejtli's 2004 paper "Past, Present, and Future of Cyclodextrin Research"; Moneek Madra and Stephen Sturley's 2010 paper "Niemann-Pick Type C Pathogenesis and Treatment: From Statins to Sugars"; and Benny Liu's 2012 review "Therapeutic Potential of Cyclodextrins in the Treatment of Niemann-Pick Type C Disease" were very helpful in understanding the history of NPC drug development. Descriptions about the February 24, 2009, meeting in New York are based on author notes from the meeting. Chris and Hugh Hempel recounted to me their experiences of the girls' first cyclodextrin infusions. It was also helpful to view the footage of the event filmed as part of the *Dateline NBC* story, "A Mom's Quest: Saving Her Twin Daughters' Lives," which aired on June 28, 2009.

77 **Scientists at the University:** Benny Liu et al., "Genetic Variations and Treatments That Affect the Lifespan of the NPC1 Mouse," *Journal of Lipid Research* 49, no. 3 (March 2008): 663–69, https:// doi.org/10.1194/jlr.M700525-JLR200.

78 **The new study:** Cristin D. Davidson et al., "Chronic Cyclodextrin Treatment of Murine Niemann-Pick C Disease Ameliorates Neuronal Cholesterol and Glycosphingolipid Storage and Disease Progression," *PLOS One* 4, no. 9 (September 2009): e6951, https://doi.org/10.1371/journal.pone.0006951.

78 **The scientists then hypothesized:** Synthia H. Mellon, Wenhui Gong, and Marcus D. Schonemann, "Endogenous and Synthetic Neurosteroids in Treatment of Niemann-Pick Type C Disease," *Brain Research Reviews* 57, no. 2 (March 2008): 410–20, https:// doi.org/10.1016/j.brainresrev.2007.05.012.

87 **This time, she wrote:** Chris Hempel, "Dear Johnson & Johnson,

Do Kids Really Matter to You?," *Addi & Cassi Fund* (blog), February 12, 2009, http://addiandcassi.com/index.php?s=dear +johnson+and+johnson.

7. NEW HIT

Events in this chapter are based on author notes from the November 13 and 14, 2009, meeting at the NIH and interviews with the parents and scientists. Chris and Hugh Hempel described cutting Chris's hair in author interviews, including on October 2, 2009, and November 16, 2009.

8. REVERBERATIONS

All descriptions of the events at the hearing are from the author's notes from the January 12, 2010 advisory committee hearing. Phil Marella's speech to the FDA was reprinted in the *Greenwich Time*, https://www.greenwichtime.com/news/article/A-plea-for-support -Phil-Marella-addresses-FDA-438929.php#page-1.

110 **In fact, a couple:** Kevin Grogan, "FDA Rejects Actelion's Zavesca for Rare NP-C Disease," *PharmaTimes Online*, February 12, 2009, https://www.pharmatimes.com/news/fda_rejects_actelions _zavesca_for_rare_np-c_disease_981662.

9. PERSUASION

Descriptions about the conference and quotes are from the author's notes from the workshop.

My article describing some of the events, "Push to Cure Rare Diseases," ran in *The Wall Street Journal* on March 10, 2010 and can be found at https://www.wsj.com/articles/SB100014240527487041 45904575111943356541152.

116 **Chris decided to:** Chris Hempel, "Update: Orphan Drug Application (Hydroxy Propel Beta Cyclodextrin)," *Global Genes* (blog), May 17, 2010, http://addiandcassi.com/fda-grants-orphan -drug-status-for-cyclodextrin-compound-to-treat-fatal-genetic -cholesterol-disease.

122 **Chris Hempel didn't:** Chris Hempel, email to Denny Porter, July 29, 2011, shared with the author.

10. THE GREATER GOOD

Denny Porter's description of his worries about the trial are from an author interview on February 12, 2013. Descriptions of Dillon's experience in the trial are based on author notes at the NIH on February 12, 2013, and interviews with the Papiers, including on July 21, 2013. The description of the meeting with the ethicists is based on author notes from the visit.

11. COMPLICATIONS

Descriptions about Cassi's surgery are based on interviews with Chris and Hugh Hempel and emails between the Hempels and Denny Porter on April 10 and April 11, 2013. Descriptions about Dillon's experience in the trial are from author interview with Darrile Papier, July 21, 2013. Descriptions of Dana Marella's funeral on July 16, 2013, are from author notes and interview with Phil and Andrea Marella at their home on August 26, 2013.

12. THE COMMUNITY'S DRUG

Information in the chapter are from author notes of the August 2013 National Niemann-Pick Disease Foundation meeting and from author interview with Andrew Mulberg, November 22, 2021.

159 **Years later, after:** Nathan Denton et al., "Data Silos Are Undermining Drug Development and Failing Rare Disease Patients," *Orphanet Journal of Rare Diseases* 161 (April 2021), https://doi.org/10.1186/s13023-021-01806-4.

161 **When Denny and Liz:** Daniel Ory et al., "Intrathecal 2-hydroxypropyl-β-cyclodextrin Decreases Neurological Disease Progression in Niemann-Pick Disease, Type C1: A Non-Randomised, Open-Label, Phase 1-2 Trial," *The Lancet* 390, no. 10104 (October 2017): 1758–68, https://doi.org/10.1016/S0140-6736(17)31465-4.

13. LILIES AND DOVES

Information in the chapter is based on author visit to Porter home on June 25, 2016; author interviews with Denny Porter and the Papiers at the National Niemann-Pick Disease Foundation meeting in Boston, Massachusetts, on August 12–14, 2016; and author notes of the Hempel family's doctor visits in Oakland, California, in June 2016. The author watched a livestream of the patient-focused drug development meeting on March 18, 2019, and interviewed Chris Hempel and other parents who attended. Descriptions of the ceremony at the Hempel home celebrating the lives of Addi and Cassi are based on author notes from the September 2019 event.

163 **The NIH signed:** Amy Dockser Marcus, "Small Biotech Gets Rights to Rare Disease Drug," *The Wall Street Journal*, January 7, 2015, https://www.wsj.com/articles/small-biotech-vtesse-gets-rights-to-rare-disease-drug-1420606861.

170 **He died at:** "Dillon Papier Obituary," *The Washington Post*, April 8, 2017, accessed March 11, 2022, https://www.legacy.com/us/obituaries/washingtonpost/name/dillon-papier-obituary?id=6081035.

170 **Dillon was one:** "Memorials," National Niemann-Pick Disease Foundation, accessed June 20, 2022, https://nnpdf.org/family-support/memorials.

171 **Phil Marella and some:** Steven U. Walkley et al., "Fostering Collaborative Research for a Rare Genetic Disease: The Example of Niemann-Pick Type C Disease," *Orphanet Journal of Rare Diseases* 11, no. 1 (2016): 161, https://doi.org/10.1186/s13023-016-0540-x.

172 **Sucampo was so:** "Sucampo Acquires Vtesse Inc.," *GlobeNewswire*, April 3, 2017, https://www.globenewswire.com/news-release/2017/04/03/953426/0/en/Sucampo-Acquires-Vtesse-Inc.html.

172 **At the National:** Amy Dockser Marcus, "For a Rare Disease, Drug Trials Scramble for Patients," *The Wall Street Journal*, August 19, 2015, https://www.wsj.com/articles/for-a-rare-disease-drug-trials-scramble-for-patients-1440013683.

14. THE CATHEDRAL OF SCIENCE

Chris Austin's quotes are from author interviews, including on October 24, 2021. Information about the Long Covid advocacy movement are from author interviews with Elisa Perego on October 24, 2021; Felicity Callard on October 26, 2021; and Hannah Wei and Lisa McCorkell on April 26, 2022. Jodi Halpern's quotes are from an author interview on April 25, 2022. Helen Burstin's quotes are from author interview on January 13, 2021. Descriptions of the NPC community meeting with Mallinckrodt officials about the cyclodextrin program are based on author notes from the January 22, 2021, meeting.

183 **He asked his:** Raymond Carver, *Cathedral: Stories* (New York: Vintage Books, 1989), 223.

184 **"Put some people":** Carver, *Cathedral*, 227.

185 **The scientists enthusiastically:** Jodi Halpern et al., "How Scien-

tists Perceive CRISPR's Translational Promise and the Implications for Individuals with Genetic Conditions," *Ethics & Human Research* 43, no. 6 (November 2021): 28–41, https://doi.org/10.1002/eahr.500108.

186 **She shared her:** Sebastian Zimmer et al., "Cyclodextrin Promotes Atherosclerosis Regression via Macrophage Reprogramming," *Science Translational Medicine* 8, no. 333 (May 2016): 333ra50, https://dx.doi.org/10.1126%2Fscitranslmed.aad6100.

187 **And when Mallinckrodt:** Amy Dockser Marcus, "When Drug Development for Rare Disease Hit Setback, Parents Were Stung," *The Wall Street Journal,* January 28, 2021, https://www.wsj.com/articles/when-drug-development-for-rare-disease-hit-setback-parents-were-stung-11611851932.

187 **But in an August:** Letter provided to the author.

188 **In a meeting:** Effy Vayena et al., "Research Led by Participants: A New Social Contract for a New Kind of Research," *Journal of Medical Ethics* 42, no. 4 (April 2016): 216–19, https://dx.doi.org/10.1136%2Fmedethics-2015-102663.

190 **The FDA stated:** "Expanded Access to Investigational Drugs for Treatment Use—Questions and Answers: Guidance for Industry," U.S. Department of Health and Human Services, Food and Drug Administration, Center for Drug Evaluation and Research (CDER), Center for Biologics Evaluation and Research (CBER), June 2016, updated October 2017, https://www.fda.gov/media/85675/download, 2.

192 **Covid patients met:** Amy Dockser Marcus, "Covid-19 Patients Are Doing Their Own Research," *The Wall Street Journal,* January 30, 2021, https://www.wsj.com/articles/covid-19-patients-are-doing-their-own-research-11611982860.

196 **He called the work:** Matt Might, "The Algorithm for Precision Medicine," bertrand.might.net, accessed March 10, 2022, https://bertrand.might.net/articles/algorithm-for-precision-medicine.

INDEX